DIAGNOSTIC PI

CLINICAL NEUROLOGY

Malcolm Parsons
MA, FRCP

Consultant Neurologist,
The General Infirmary at Leeds and
Pinderfields Hospital, Wakefield.
Senior Lecturer in Clinical Neurology at
The University of Leeds, England.

Wolfe Medical Publications Ltd

Titles in this series, published or being developed, include:

Diagnostic Picture Tests in Paediatrics

Picture Tests in Human Anatomy

Diagnostic Picture Tests in Oral Medicine

Diagnostic Picture Tests in Orthopaedics

Diagnostic Picture Tests in Infectious Diseases

Diagnostic Picture Tests in Dermatology

Diagnostic Picture Tests in Ophthalmology

Diagnostic Picture Tests in Rheumatology

Diagnostic Picture Tests in Obstetrics/Gynaecology

Diagnostic Picture Tests in Clinical Neurology

Diagnostic Picture Tests in Injury in Sport

Diagnostic Picture Tests in Surgery

Diagnostic Picture Tests in General Medicine

Copyright © M. Parsons, 1987
Published by Wolfe Medical Publications Ltd. 1987
Printed by W.S. Cowell Ltd, Ipswich, England
ISBN 0 7234 0919 6

For a full list of Wolfe Medical Atlases, plus
forthcoming titles and details of our surgical,
dental and veterinary Atlases, please write to
Wolfe Medical Publications Limited,
Wolfe House,
3 Conway Street,
London W1P 6HE

Preface

This book is designed to help those preparing for examinations to test their knowledge of neurology. It touches on most aspects of the subject but concentrates on those which lend themselves to illustration. To simulate examination conditions I have deliberately avoided a systematic layout but readers will often find that the clinical features, radiology and anatomy of a topic are dealt with in sequence.

I was asked by the publisher to grade the questions so that the first section is usually within the scope of an MB candidate, and to keep the answers short. These tasks, as those who try to concoct their own entries for half a dozen illustrations will find, are not easy. In particular, it is virtually impossible to give concise and indisputable answers to any but the most mundane questions. I hope, however, that readers will agree with the tenor of those given, but if an indignant student is driven back to his books that is no bad thing.

I would like to thank the numerous colleagues who have allowed me to examine their patients, and the photographers and technicians whose work is reproduced, Dr M. Nelson who reviewed the X-rays, Miss R. Bailey who drew the illustrations, and my wife who typed the manuscript. Above all, I thank the patients who, by allowing themselves to be photographed, made the production of the book possible.

For Clare

He who hears, forgets;
he who sees, remembers;
he who does, knows.

(Chinese proverb)

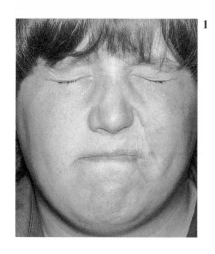

1, 2 (a) What is the matter with this man's face?
(b) What is the cause, and what associated condition sometimes develops for the same reason?
(c) What treatment would you advise?

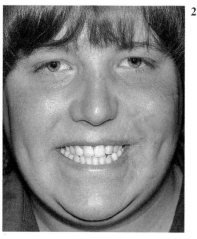

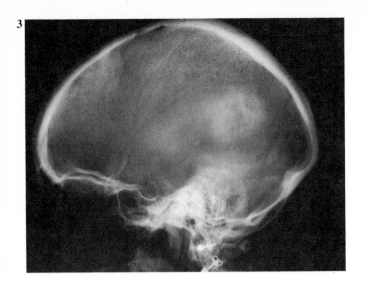

3, 4 (a) What are the main abnormalities shown on these films?
(b) What is the most likely diagnosis?
(c) How would such a patient present?

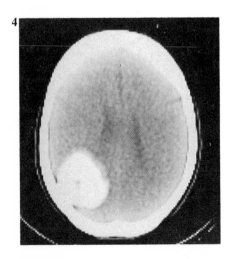

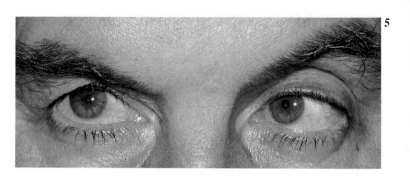

5 An elderly man suddenly developed diplopia on looking to the right.
(a) What is the matter with his eyes?
(b) If he covers his right eye, which of the two images will disappear?
(c) How extensively should he be investigated?

6 (a) Which nerve(s) supply the area affected by this naevus?
(b) Which other clinical features would you look for?
(c) What is the name and the pathology of the syndrome you suspect?

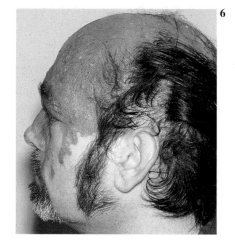

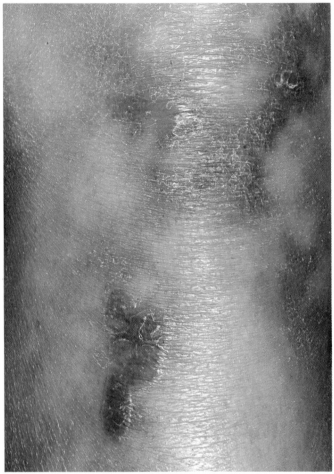

7 A patient with tuberculosis developed blisters on the legs.
(a) What is the likely diagnosis?
(b) What is the cause?
(c) Which other neurological conditions are produced in the same way?

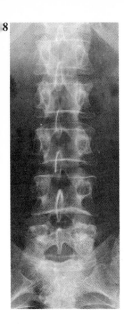
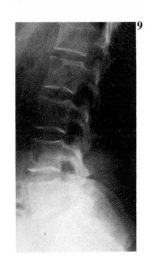

8, 9 This patient presented with a spastic paraplegia.
(a) What is the relevance of these X-rays?
(b) What is the lowest limit of the spinal cord in an adult; in a child; of the dural sac?

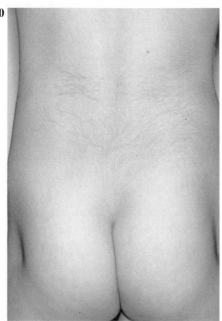

10, 11 An 11-year-old girl, treated for talipes calcaneus in infancy, complained of a limp and inability to run.
(a) What do the illustrations suggest?
(b) What would you look for?
(c) How should she be managed?

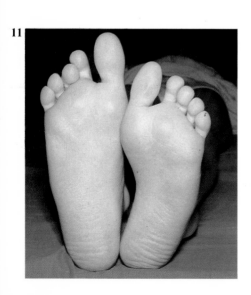

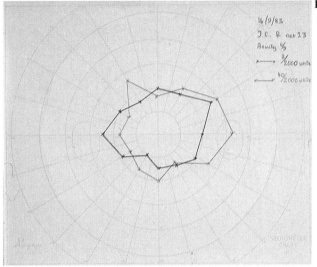

12 (a) What is used to do this test, and what is being tested?
(b) What does this result indicate?
(c) What other abnormalities might the investigation show in such a patient?

13 (a) What does this scan show?
(b) On which cranial nerves are such lesions most commonly found?

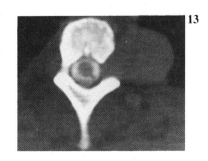

14 (a) What are these lesions?
(b) Suggest two ways in which such a patient could present as a neurological emergency.
(c) What is the unusual abnormality sometimes found in the CSF?

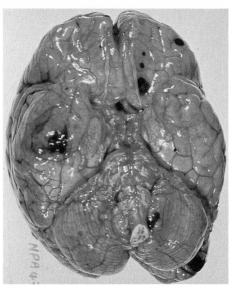

15 A young woman complained of weakness of the right arm after a brief but very intense bout of pain in the right shoulder.
(a) What does the illustration show, and what is the cause?
(b) What is the likely diagnosis?
(c) What is the prognosis?

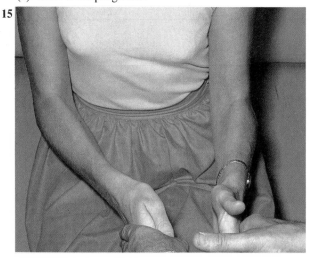

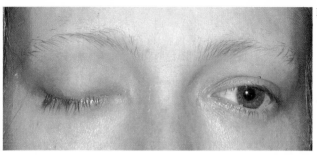

16 (a) What is the most likely anatomical cause of this lesion?
(b) What might be seen if the eyelid were raised?
(c) Which other conditions sometimes produce a similar picture?

17 (a) Which view is this and what does it show?
(b) What signs might be found with such a lesion?
(c) What other disability might the patient have?

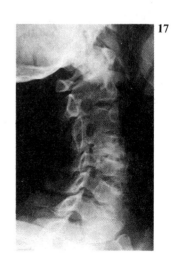

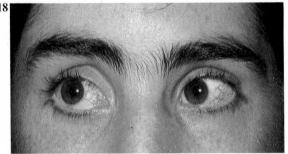

18 This child, like his siblings, was said to be unsteady on his feet.
(a) What is the diagnosis?
(b) What abnormalities would you look for in the blood?
(c) What are the likely causes of death?

19 (a) What is this?
(b) With what clinical condition is it associated?
(c) Are the patient's children likely to be affected?

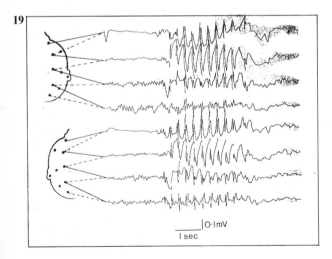

0·1mV

1 sec

20 An X-ray of the knee of a patient with epilepsy.
(a) What is the diagnosis?
(b) Which aspect of the social history would you explore?
(c) Which other neurological complications occur?

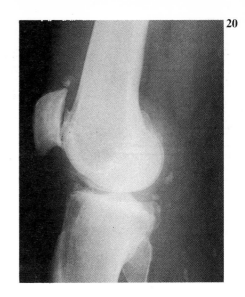

21 (a) What is a myopathy; a myelopathy; a muscular dystrophy?
(b) Which characteristic features of a muscular dystrophy are illustrated?

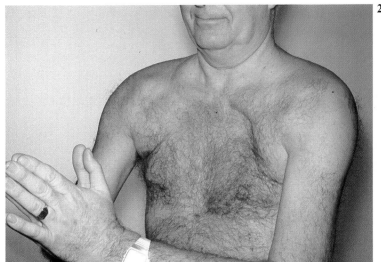

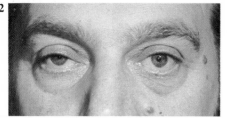

22 A 50-year-old man with no previous history of headache complained of severe and protracted R retro-orbital pain. Signs were as shown; the face perspired normally.
(a) What does the illustration show?
(b) Where is the lesion?
(c) What is the syndrome called?

23 (a) What is used to do this test, and what is being tested?
(b) What does the result suggest?
(c) Is the patient fit to drive?

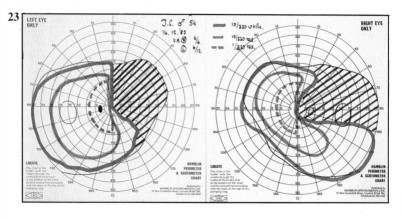

24 A man complained of bouts of severe but short-lived pain in his legs.
(a) What is illustrated?
(b) What diagnosis should be considered?
(c) Which other (possible) manifestation of this disease is present?

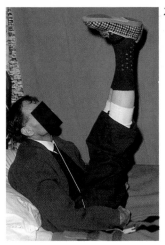

25 (a) What are the structures marked and the abnormalities shown?
(b) How do such lesions present?
(c) How are they treated?

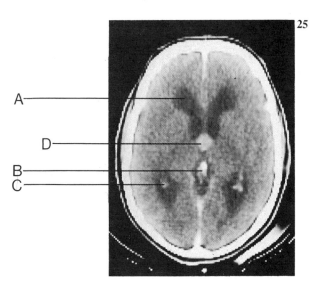

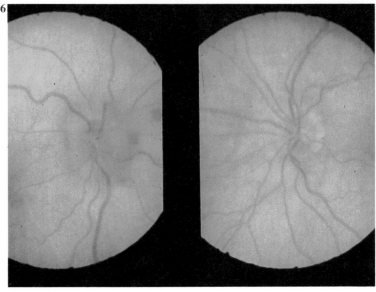

26 A 69-year-old man became forgetful and unsteady on his feet over the course of a year.
(a) What is the abnormality shown?
(b) What is the likely cause?
(c) For which other sign would you look?

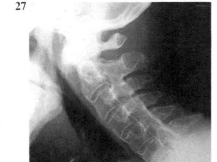

27 (a) What is the diagnosis?
(b) What are the main neurological complications in this condition?
(c) What are the main neuropathological findings?

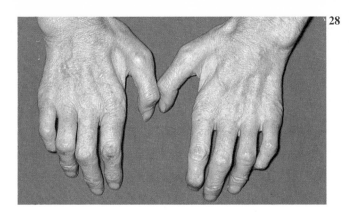

28 (a) What are the two best known neurological causes of this condition?
(b) How are they distinguished clinically?
(c) Name other possible causes.

29 (a) What is the segmental value of this sensory level?
(b) What clinical features would confirm that the level gives a true indication of the site of the lesion?
(c) How could a lesion below this point produce this level?

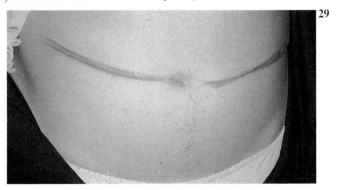

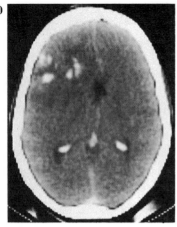

30 A right-handed woman with a 6-month history of attacks in which the right side of her face and neck felt warm and she was unable to express what she wanted to say.
(a) What is being described?
(b) Which other symptoms would you enquire about?
(c) What is illustrated?

31 The neck of a 40-year-old woman who, like her brother, had peripheral neuritis.
(a) What is the most likely diagnosis?
(b) Which other neurological signs would you look for?
(c) What is the cause?

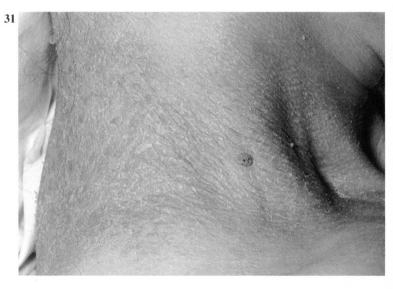

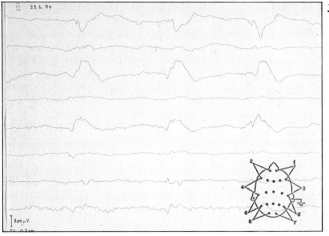

32 A 60-year-old woman with a 5-day history of malaise leading on to confusion and drowsiness.
(a) What does the illustration show?
(b) What is the diagnosis?
(c) What is your definition of this group of diseases?

33 (a) What is the main abnormality shown on this film?
(b) What would be the next investigation?
(c) Which nerves might be damaged by such a lesion?

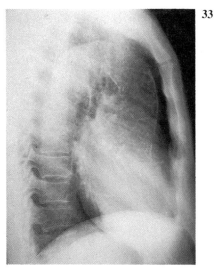

33

34 A man attended for a routine medical examination.

(a) What diagnosis does his appearance suggest?

(b) Which two neurological abnormalities are most likely to be found on examination?

(c) What treatment would you advise?

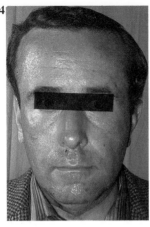

35 This lady complained of an unpleasant alteration in sensation in the area indicated.

(a) What is its innervation?

(b) Can you suggest a cause?

(c) What is this condition called?

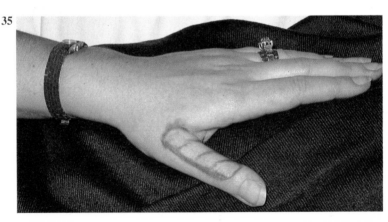

36 A 78-year-old woman complained of severe pain in the R ear. She was said to have cervical spondylosis and her R shoulder was weak.
(a) What does the film show?
(b) What is the likely diagnosis?
(c) What caused her earache?

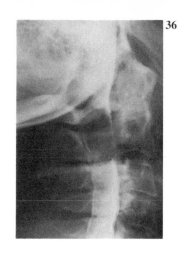

37 A 45-year-old man with a family history of weakness in the limbs.
(a) What is illustrated, and what is the most likely cause?
(b) Which other muscles in the upper limb are most likely to be affected?
(c) Which other hereditary conditions can produce a similar picture?

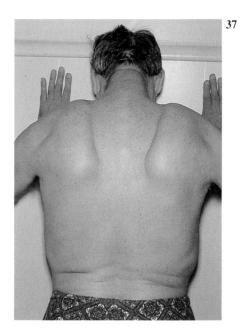

38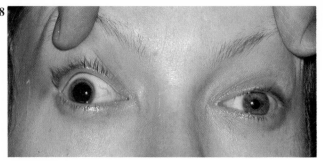

38–41 (a) What is the matter with this patient?
(b) Is the trochlear nerve functioning normally?
(c) What is the most likely cause of the trouble?

39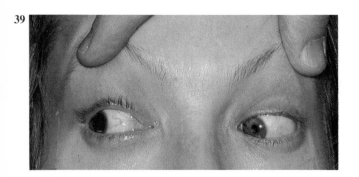

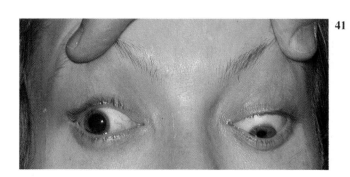

40

41

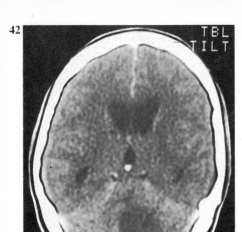

42 This man's brother had a cerebellar tumour.

(a) What does the film show?

(b) How do such lesions present?

(c) What other abnormalities would you look for?

43 (a) What is a fit?

(b) Would you prescribe anticonvulsants for this patient?

(c) Name two other important measures that might be taken.

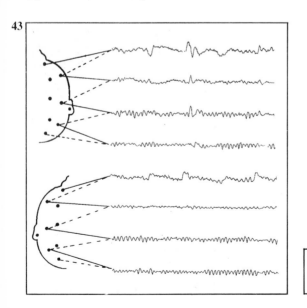

0·1mV

1 sec

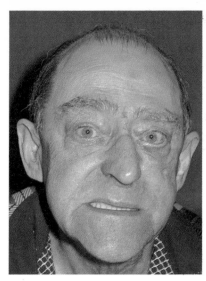

44, 45 (a) What is illustrated?
(b) What are the likely causes?

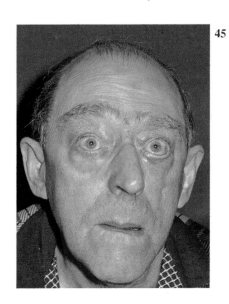

46 (a) What does this X-ray show?
(b) What is the likely diagnosis?

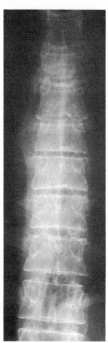

47 (a) What does this section show?
(b) What are the cardinal features of this condition?
(c) What abnormalities are found in the CSF?

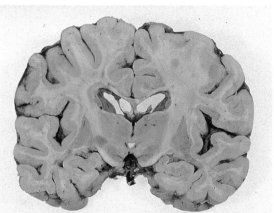

TEST-TYPES.

N.5

But the accident that followed, though it be a trifle, will be very diverting in its place. I was exceedingly diverted with this journey. I found in the low grounds hares, as I thought them to be, and foxes; but they differed greatly from all the other kinds I had met with, nor could I satisfy myself to eat them, though I killed several. But I had no need to be venturous, for I had no want of food, and that which was very good too, especially these three sorts, viz., goats, pigeons, and turtle, or tortoise; which, added to my grapes, Leadenhall Market could not have furnished a table better than I, in proportion to the company. And though my case was deplorable enough, yet I had great cause for thankfulness, and that I was not driven to any extremities for food, but rather plenty, even to dainties. I never travelled in this journey above two miles outright in a day, or thereabouts;
car swim marine ear nurse crane economic sun

N.6

with a row of stakes, set upright in the ground, either from one tree to another, or so as no wild creature could come at me without waking me. As soon as I came to the seashore, I was surprised to see that I had taken up my lot on the worst side of the island, for here indeed the shore was covered with innumerable turtles; whereas, on the other side, I found but three in a year and a half. Here was also an infinite number of fowls of many kinds, some of which I had seen, and some which I had not seen before, and many of them very good meat, but such as I knew not the names of, except those called penguins. I could have shot as many as I pleased, but was very sparing of my ruin cove examine rain swan ease conserve move

N.8

of the island, yet it was with much more difficulty that I could come near them, the country being flat and even, and they saw me much sooner than when I was on the hill. I confess this side of the country was much pleasanter than mine; but yet I had not the least inclination to remove, for as I was fixed in my habitation, it became natural to me, and I seemed all the while I was here to be as it were upon a journey, and from home. However, I travelled along the shore of the sea towards the east, I suppose about twelve miles, and then setting up a great pole nave rim common assess rinse swarm cocoon car

48 (a) For what is this test-type used?
(b) What should the patient be asked to do before using it?
(c) What score would be expected in a patient who can read 6/18 on a Snellen chart?

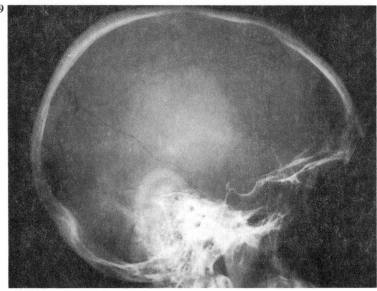

49, 50 (a) What do these illustrations show?
(b) What is the usual cause of this lesion?
(c) How characteristic is the 'lucid interval'?

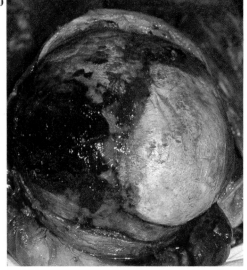

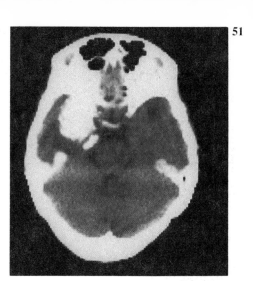

51 (a) What does this unenhanced scan show?
(b) What is the lesion?
(c) How would it present?

52 (a) What does this chart demonstrate?
(b) What is the likely cause?
(c) What is the prognosis?

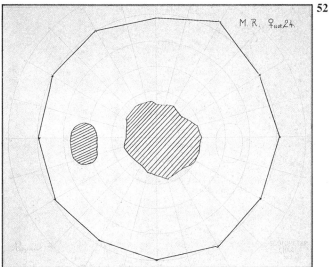

53

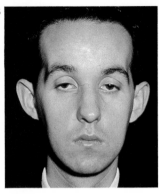

53 (a) What is the matter with this man's eyes?
(b) Which conditions commonly produce such an abnormality?
(c) What is the diagnosis?

54 A 55-year-old patient with ptosis, diplopia, dysphagia and weakness of the shoulders.
(a) What is the diagnosis and what is the lesion?
(b) Should it be removed and, if so, why?
(c) Is a change in medical treatment likely to be required in the immediate postoperative period?

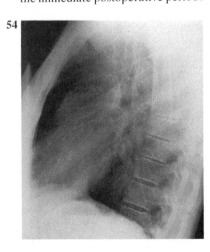

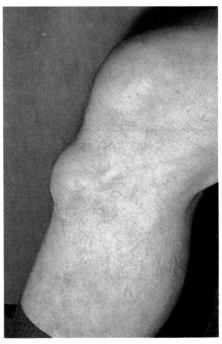

55, 56 These lesions were found on a man aged 50 years.
(a) What are they, and what is the diagnosis?
(b) For which other manifestations of this condition would you look?
(c) Is there an enhanced risk of neurological disease?

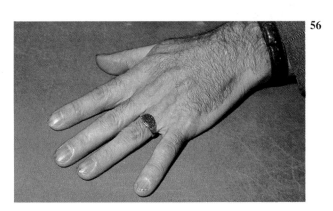

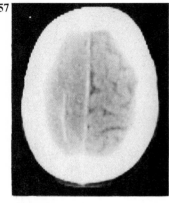

57 (a) What does this scan show?
(b) What is the cause of such lesions?
(c) What is the most common sign?

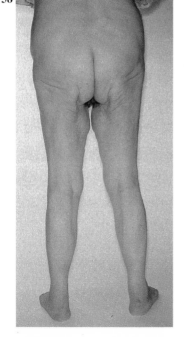

58 A 58-year-old diabetic with a 6-month history of pain and weakness in the hips and the R thigh. The R quadriceps were wasted and the knee jerks were absent, but sensation and bladder control were normal.
(a) What does the illustration show?
(b) What diagnosis does this story suggest?
(c) What are the aetiology and prognosis?

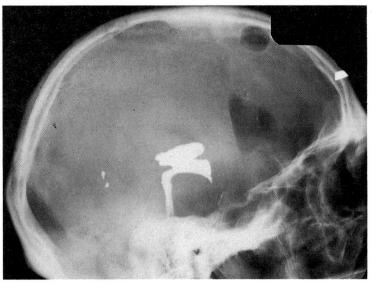

59 (a) What does this X-ray show?
(b) Where is the lesion?
(c) What is the eponym of this radiological sign?

60 (a) What is the most likely diagnosis?
(b) For which other neurological signs would you look?
(c) Which form of the disease is this?

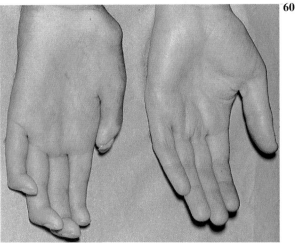

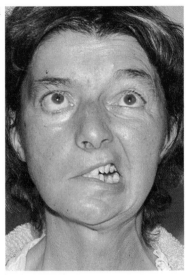

61, 62 (a) What is the abnormality shown in **61**?
(b) In **62** the patient is trying to look to the right. Where is the lesion?
(c) What are the most likely causes?

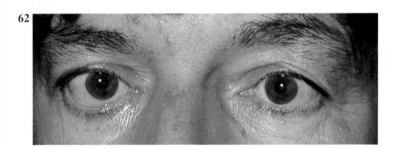

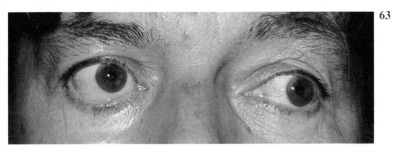

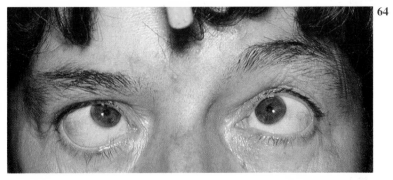

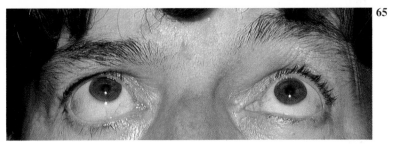

63–65 (a) What is this abnormality?
(b) Where is the lesion?
(c) This is the patient shown in **61** and **62**. What is the name of the ocular syndrome?

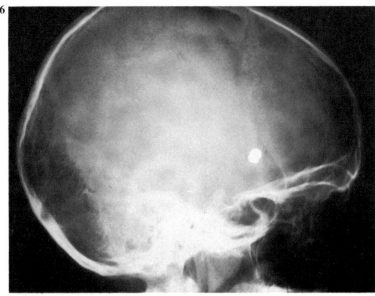

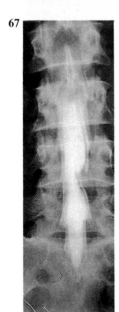

66 A child with an airgun slug in his brain had one fit shortly after admission.
(a) Would you prescribe anticonvulsants i) at once ii) long-term?
(b) What other complication might occur?

67 (a) What does this X-ray show, and what is the likely cause?
(b) Describe the abnormality in detail.
(c) Which neurological signs might be expected?

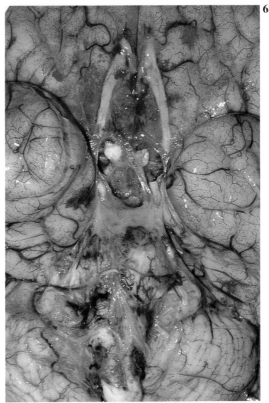

68 A 9-year-old child complained of ear-ache for a few days and then, over 24 hours, lapsed into coma.
(a) What is the diagnosis?
(b) What advice would you give to a practitioner requesting admission of such a case?
(c) Would you perform a lumbar puncture?

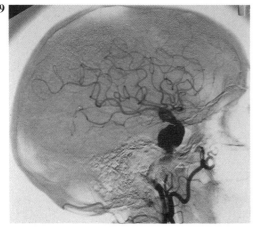

69, 70 (a) What is this lesion?
(b) Which nerves could it damage?
(c) What will be the appearance of the pupil?

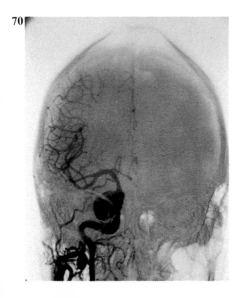

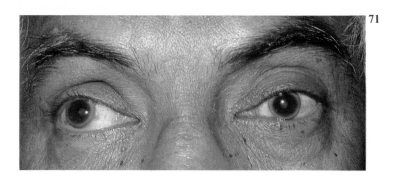

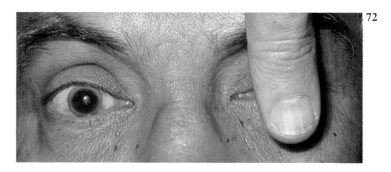

71, 72 The cover test helps to distinguish between two sorts of squint.
(a) What are they?
(b) How does it distinguish between them?
(c) How else do they differ?

73

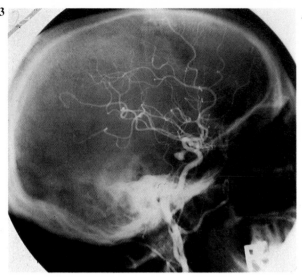

73 (a) What abnormality does this film show?
(b) How is such a patient likely to present?

74 (a) What is the matter with this patient?
(b) What are the three main commonly accepted causes of
this condition?
(c) What is MPTP?

74

A. B. C. DE FGHI JKLMNOPQR ST UVWXYZ

75 A 60-year-old man suddenly developed headache, vomiting and ataxia.
(a) What does this unenhanced scan show, and what is the likely cause?
(b) What is the treatment?

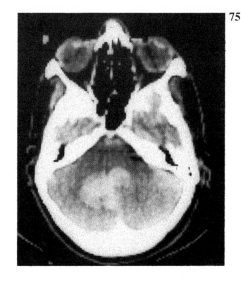

76 This man discovered that vision in his L eye was seriously impaired when, after a minor injury, the R eye was occluded.
(a) What is the matter with the fundus?
(b) Which other ocular abnormalities would you look for?
(c) What does the history suggest?

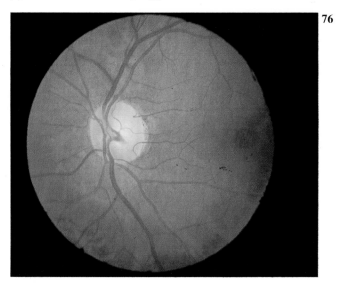

77

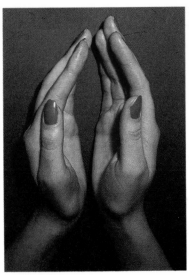

77 (a) What does this illustration show, and what is the commonest cause of such a defect?
(b) In what respects is the picture atypical, and can you think of another explanation?

78

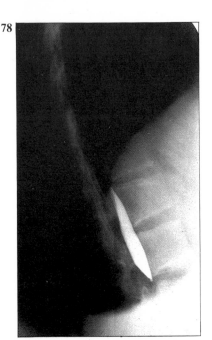

78 A young man developed severe lumbago followed by numbness and weakness in the legs soon after a minor injury to his back. He had a white cell count of 37,000, but had recently had a boil on his face.
(a) What diagnosis does this film—taken in a head-down position—suggest?
(b) What is the treatment?
(c) What precaution should be taken when performing a lumbar puncture?

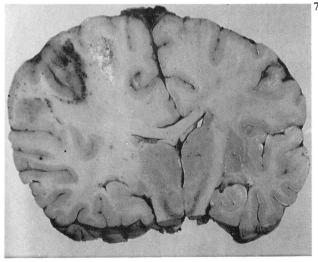

79 (a) What does this illustration show?
(b) What are the presenting features of such a lesion?
(c) Name some potential causes.

80 Examination of a motorist found unconscious at the wheel of her car after a minor accident revealed this lesion.
(a) What is it?
(b) Should she have been driving?
(c) Is she liable to be prosecuted?

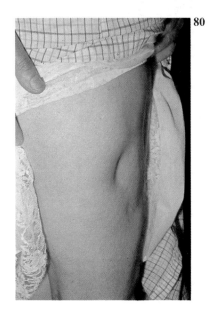

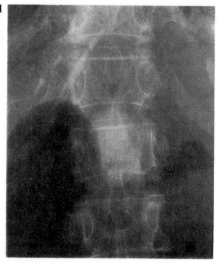

81, 82 (a) What do these films show?
(b) What is the likely diagnosis?
(c) What are the indications for Queckenstedt's test?

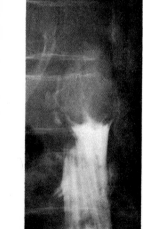

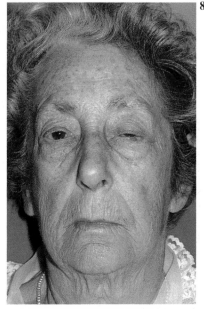

83

83, 84 These photographs were taken one minute apart.
(a) What is the diagnosis, and what has been done?
(b) What other investigations should be carried out?
(c) Which drug occasionally produces a similar condition?

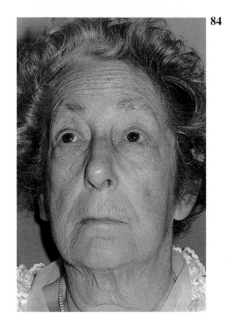

84

85

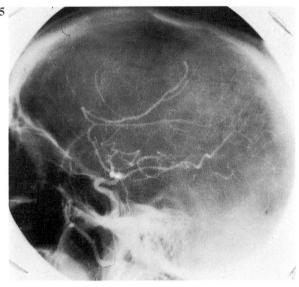

85 (a) What does this film show?
(b) How might such a patient present?
(c) What would you look for on the skull X-ray?

86

Two nembutal give me brief
respite from the fear. For
awhile it is dissipated, and I
can walk to the paper shop,
alone. But within an hour or
so. I slip back, imperceptably,
into the awful groove of
intense tyranny whole being
a prey to nervous tension, which
has an odd paralysing effect
on me. If only I could get
into active motion... but the
physical is affecting me so
greatly, psychologically, that
most of my waking hours
are ones of mediaval tortures.
I can only ask God to help
me until Dr. Caddy returns.
Perhaps, after I have spoken
to him, I'll regain that lost
confidence.... It MUST come
- it simply must.... I cannot.
after all the many, many years
of battling against overwhelming odds,
accept defeat. I must win through
retain as much independence as
possible, and return to my
beloved home again ...

86 (a) What is the matter with this patient?
(b) Where is the lesion?
(c) For which other signs would you look?

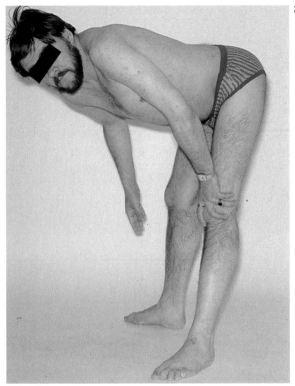

87 Gowers' sign in a patient with a family history of weakness.
(a) What does it indicate?
(b) In this instance what diagnosis does it suggest?

88

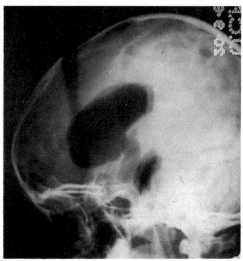

88 (a) What is the name of this investigation?
(b) What does it show?
(c) What are the likely causes of the abnormalities?

89 A young man complained of severe headaches and then developed focal fits followed by paralysis on the L. There was a tender swelling over the R temple.
(a) What is the diagnosis?
(b) What causes such lesions?
(c) What caused the fits and weakness?

89

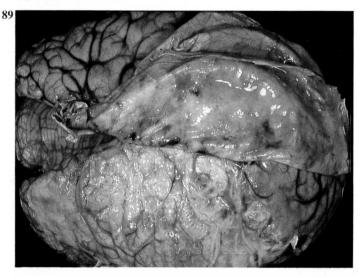

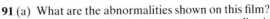

ABCDEFIJKMNOPQ:

ABCDEFIJKLHNOPQ.

Could ~~by~~ would be as for awall

90 (a) What is this condition?
(b) How do you define it?
(c) Where is the lesion?

91 (a) What are the abnormalities shown on this film?
(b) Is raised intracranial pressure a common complication?
(c) Is the condition hereditary?

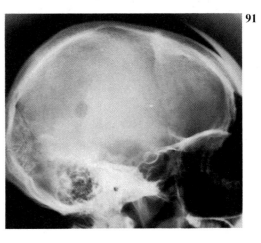

92

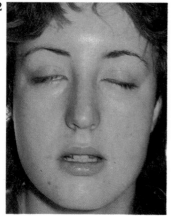

93

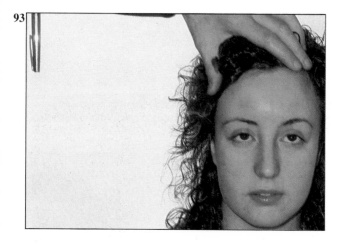

92–97 Over 7 days this woman developed diplopia, oscillopsia, ataxia, R facial weakness and numbness of the L hand. She had a bilateral internuclear ophthalmoplegia and increased reflexes on the L.
(a) Where is the lesion?
(b) What do the illustrations—taken after further deterioration—show?
(c) What is the diagnosis?

94

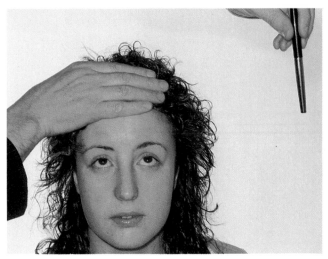

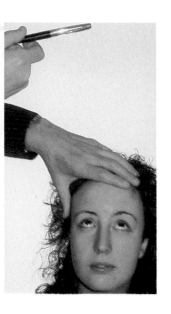

96

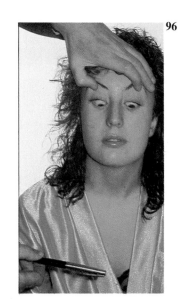

97

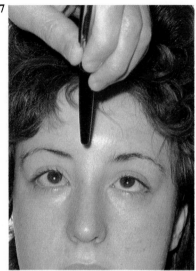

98 Two weeks before admission this elderly hypertensive man developed a severe headache, confusion and a tendency to bump into objects on the L.
(a) What does this unenhanced scan show?
(b) To what is the lesion attributable, and in what respect is it unusual?
(c) What are the treatment and prognosis?

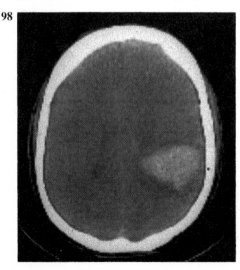

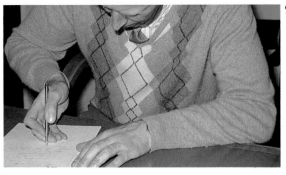

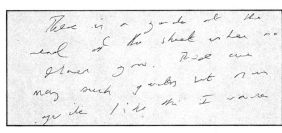

99, 100 This man's writing had deteriorated because he could no longer hold a pen correctly (**99**). Some improvement was effected by altering his grip (**100**).

(a) What would you ask him; what diagnosis do you suspect?
(b) What is the aetiology of this condition?
(c) What is the treatment?

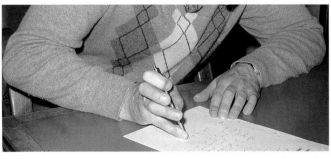

101

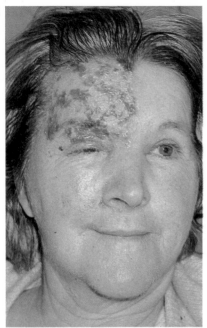

101 (a) What is this condition?
(b) What are the two most common complications?
(c) What is the aetiology?

102

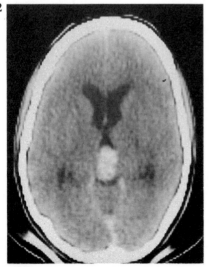

102 (a) What does this film show?
(b) What is the lesion?
(c) How would it present?

103 (a) What is the condition with which this lesion is associated?
(b) How does it arise, and what other abnormalities may be found in the vicinity?
(c) Do subsequent children run an above-average risk of having the same condition?

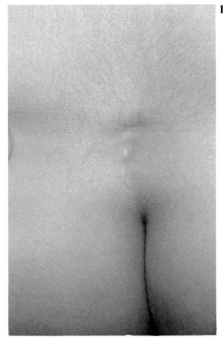

104 A patient developed a boil on his nose, followed within 24 hours by diffuse swelling on the L side of his face.
(a) What is the diagnosis?
(b) What is the most likely complication?
(c) For how long should antibiotics be given?

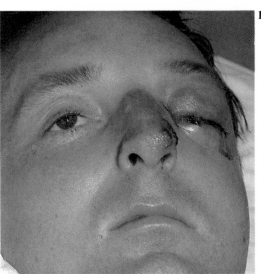

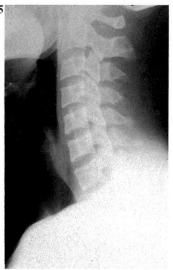 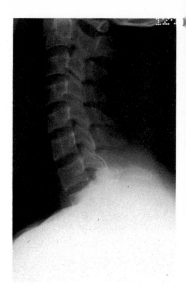

105, 106 A young Indian doctor had a short history of pain in the neck, the back of the L arm and the inner aspect of the L hand. It was aggravated by jolting. The deep flexors and intrinsic muscles were weak, the reflexes were intact and sensation over the inner aspect of the hand and forearm was impaired.
(a) Where is the lesion?
(b) How do these X-rays—taken at the same session—differ?
(c) What is your working diagnosis?

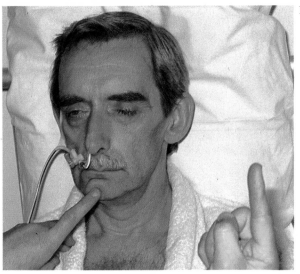

107 A 53-year-old man with a 72-hour history of diplopia, dysphonia and dysphagia. He was otherwise well.
(a) What disabilities are present?
(b) What is the diagnosis?
(c) What is the pathology?

108 A 70-year-old patient with a short history of sudden attacks of loss of consciousness. An EEG and a 24-hour ECG recording were normal, but this ECG was obtained during a subsequent attack.
(a) What does it show?
(b) What is the treatment?

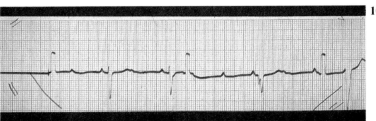

109 (a) What is the main abnormality shown?
(b) What is the 'textbook' presentation?
(c) What is the highest level of severe complications acceptable if surgery is to be beneficial?

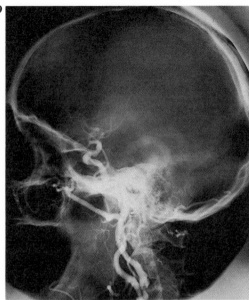

110 This woman complained of numbness, which was attributed to multiple sclerosis, in the area indicated.
(a) What is the likely diagnosis?
(b) What is the fullest extent of the disability?

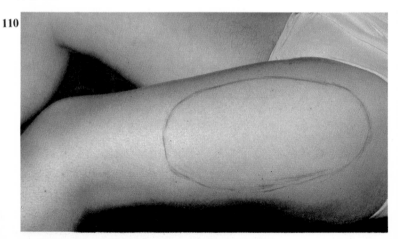

111 (a) What is the diagnosis?
(b) What is a plexiform neuroma?
(c) Which related possibilities would you consider if such a patient complained of visual failure?

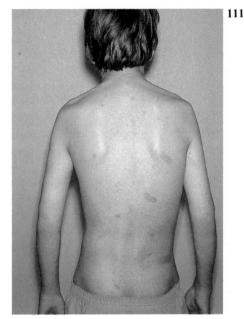

112 (a) What diagnosis does this film suggest?
(b) How do such patients present?
(c) Which of the systemic manifestations usually appears first?

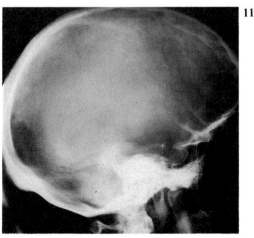

113

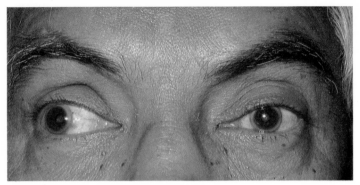

114

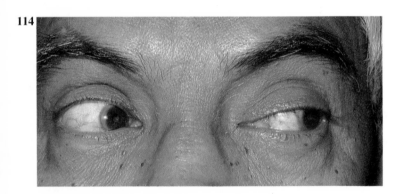

115

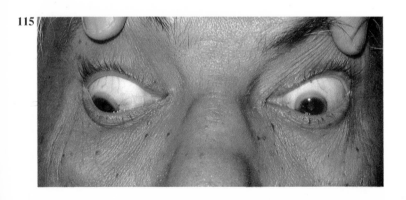

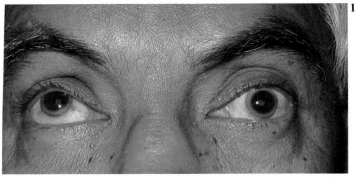

113–116 (a) What is the matter with this man?
(b) What are the most likely causes?

117 (a) What is this condition?
(b) How is it transmitted?
(c) What subdivisions of this condition are recognised?

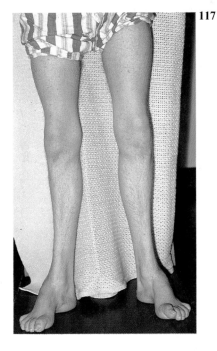

118

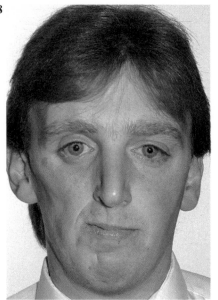

119

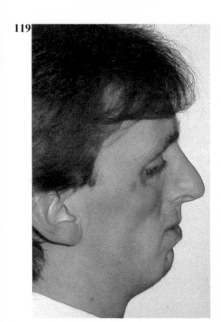

1

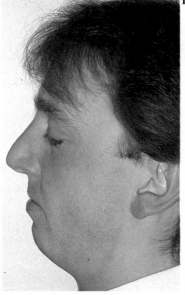

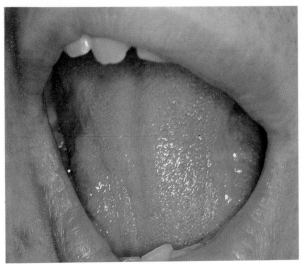

118–121 A 23-year-old man complained that the R side of his face had 'shrunk' in the previous 4 months.
(a) What is the diagnosis?
(b) What is the aetiology?
(c) What is the treatment?

122

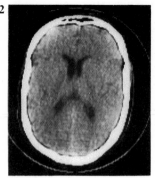 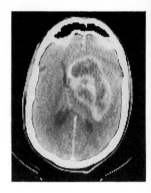

122, 123 A 57-year-old man with a 7-month history of personality change, intellectual impairment and headache. The first scan was passed as normal. The second was taken 3 months later.
(a) What does the second scan show?
(b) Would you advise surgery, radio- or chemotherapy?
(c) Not having had a fit, is he entitled to drive?

124 A diagram of the 7th nerve in the petrous temporal bone.
(a) Label 1–6.
(b) Why are 1–3 important in a patient with facial palsy?

124

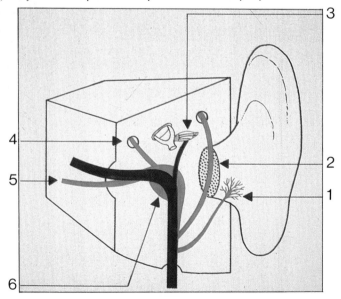

125 (a) What is this lesion?
(b) Name three conditions in which such lesions are found.
(c) To what are they attributable?

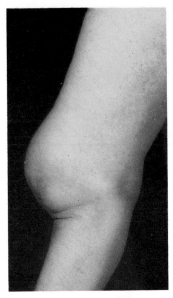

126 A woman with Parinaud's syndrome, showing loss of upward gaze and lid retraction.
(a) Which other ocular defects are closely associated with this syndrome?
(b) What are the common causes?
(c) How might upward movement of the eyes be induced?

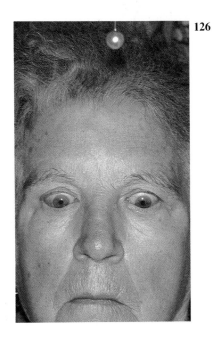

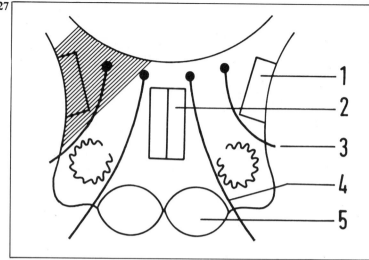

127–130 (a) Identify the structures indicated.
(b) Where do 1 and 2 join?
(c) Of what conditions are these lesions typical?
(d) What sign is common to them all?
(e) What are the other manifestations of 127?

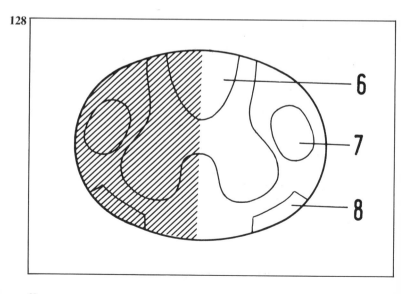

129

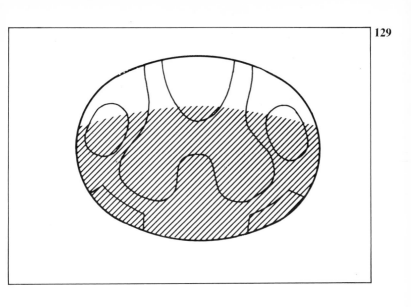

130

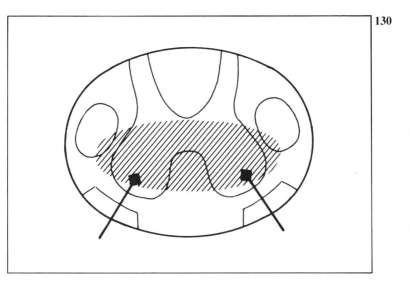

69

131

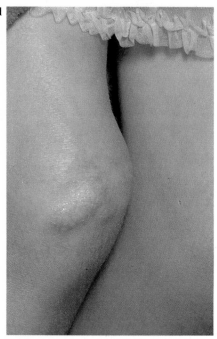

131 A 33-year-old woman, over 8 years, developed proximal weakness, nodules on knees and elbows, dysphagia, arthritis and a rash.
(a) What is the diagnosis?
(b) What are the nodules?
(c) Is she likely to have an occult carcinoma?

132

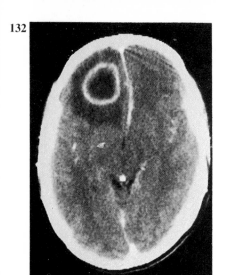

132 (a) What is this lesion?
(b) What are the common causes?
(c) Would lumbar puncture help in diagnosis or management?

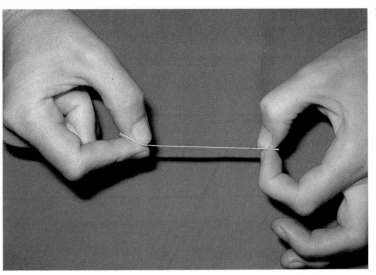

133 A young woman complained of intense but short-lived pain in the R shoulder followed by weakness in the shoulder and hand.
(a) What does the illustration demonstrate?
(b) What is the cause?

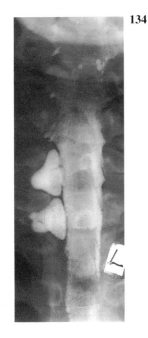

134 (a) What are these lesions, and with what are they associated?
(b) What major disability would you expect to find on examination?
(c) Which other signs would you look for and why?

135

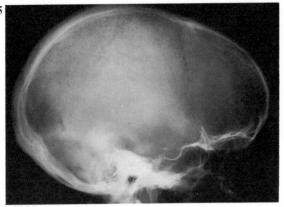

135, 136 (a) What are the main abnormalities?
(b) What lesions are commonly found in this area?
(c) How might such a patient present?

136

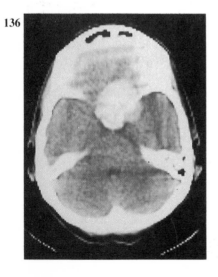

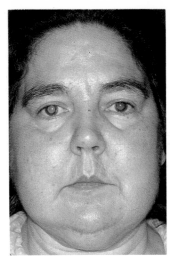

137, 138 A woman complained of headache, vomiting, diplopia and episodes of visual obscuration. Her periods were irregular and her blood pressure was normal.
(a) What is the likely diagnosis?
(b) What investigations should be ordered?
(c) What causes would you look for?

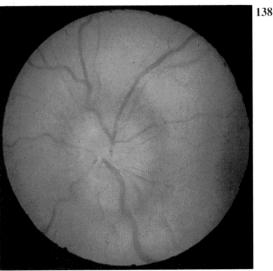

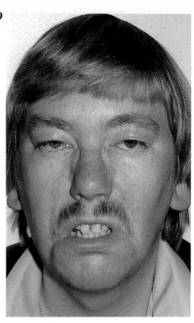

139, 140 (a) What is this congenital disorder?
(b) Which other abnormalities would you look for?
(c) Is it inherited?

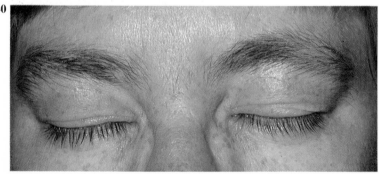

141 (a) What is this lesion?
(b) What is the usual cause of such lesions?
(c) How do isolated lesions of this sort present?

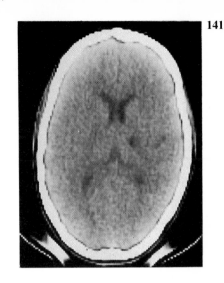

142 A 55-year-old man with intractable 'fibrositis' in the L shoulder.
(a) What does the X-ray show?
(b) What are the most likely causes?
(c) Which nerves might be damaged by such a lesion?

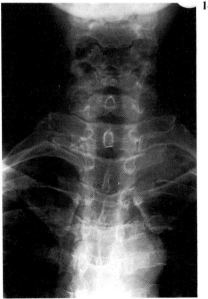

143

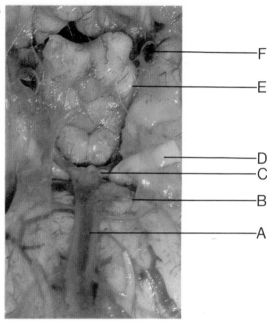

143 (a) What are the structures marked A–F?
(b) What is the main abnormality?
(c) What physical sign would you look for under these circumstances?

144

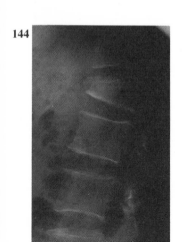

144 (a) What is the differential diagnosis?
(b) Which neurological signs would you look for?
(c) What is the anatomical basis of these signs?

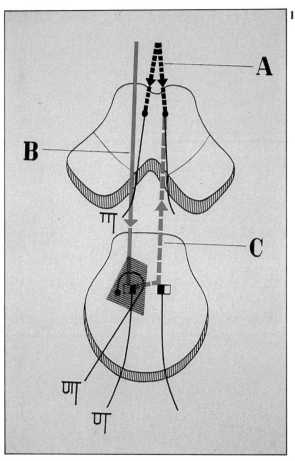

145 A diagram of the brainstem mechanism which controls ocular movements.

(a) From where do the tracts marked A and B come?

(b) What is C, and what does a lesion at this point produce?

146

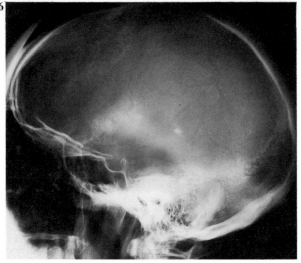

146–148 (a) What is the main abnormality shown on these films?
(b) What are the implications of this finding?

147

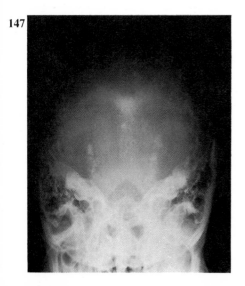

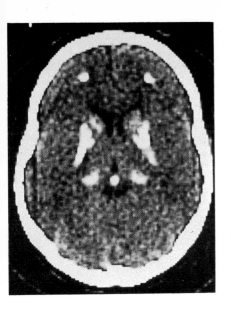

149 (a) What presenting symptoms would you expect from a tumour arising in the corpus callosum?
(b) How would you treat a patient with a lesion like this?
(c) What is the linear haemorrhagic scar on the R?

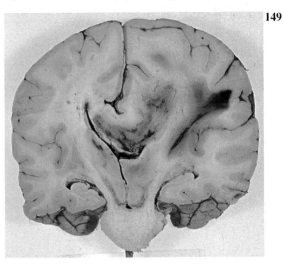

150

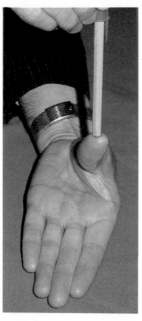

150 (a) Which muscle is being tested?
(b) What is its innervation?
(c) Which other muscle in the hand is usually supplied exclusively by this nerve?

151

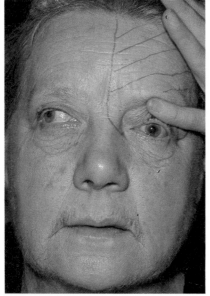

151 (a) What is shown in the illustration?
(b) Where and what is the lesion most likely to be?
(c) Which other signs would you expect?

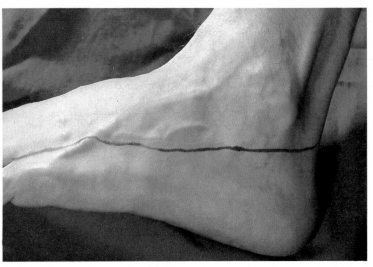

152 A 47-year-old man developed numbness and weakness in both hands and the L foot over several months.
(a) What is the abnormality illustrated?
(b) What would you ask about?
(c) Under what circumstances is such an abnormality found?

153 (a) What is this condition, and what is its aetiology?
(b) Which other neurological lesion produces a similar picture, and how would you distinguish between them?

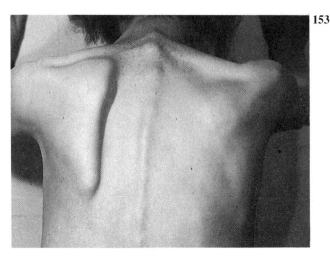

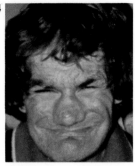

154 This long-standing epileptic man illustrates one of the side effects of treatment.
(a) What is it and what causes it?
(b) Will it get better if the drug is withdrawn?
(c) What other complications of a similar nature are described?

155 (a) What does the scan show?
(b) What is the lesion, and what symptoms is it likely to produce?

155

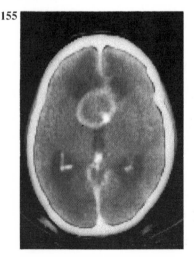

156, 157 (a) What is demonstrated in the pictures?
(b) What type of lesion do they indicate?

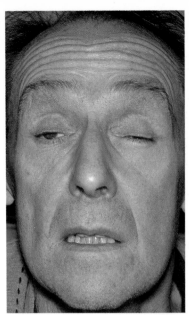

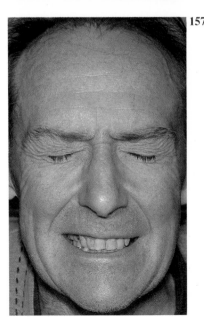

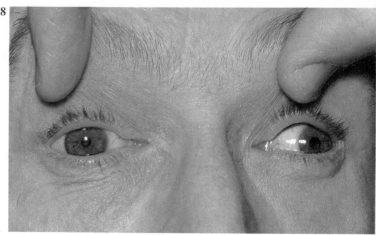

158–160 On recovery from a fit this elderly man had bilateral ptosis and diplopia (same case as **156, 157**).
(a) What do the illustrations show?
(b) Where is the lesion?
(c) Which part of this structure has (almost) escaped?

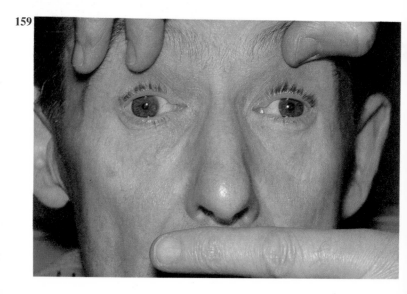

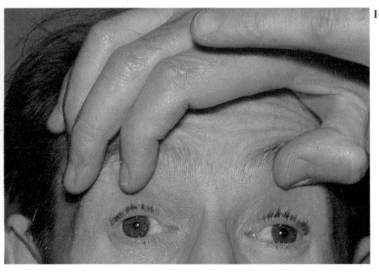

161 (a) What does this film show?
(b) What is the diagnosis?

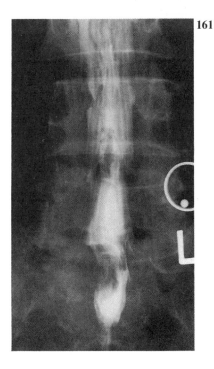

162

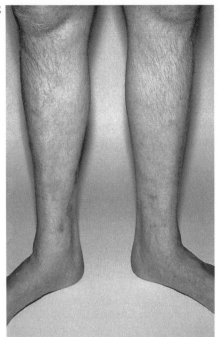

162, 163 A patient with renal failure developed 'peripheral neuritis' (ie numbness over the soles of the feet) after insertion of a shunt.
(a) What has happened?
(b) Does renal failure cause a neuropathy or a myopathy?

163

20/8 Urea ↑ ↗ 60 mmol.

   Shunt attempted in Ⓛ ankle Yesterday.

Ⓛ post. tibialis artery branching into
several small vessels.

Ⓡ post. tibialis artery ∴ used.

164 (a) What abnormality is shown on this film?
(b) When is this finding significant?
(c) Where is the lesion?

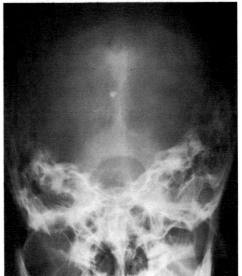

165 (a) What does this post-contrast scan show?
(b) What is the diagnosis?
(c) At what stage is this picture most likely to be seen?

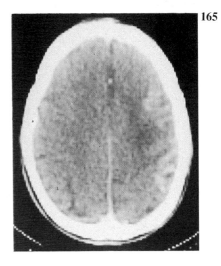

166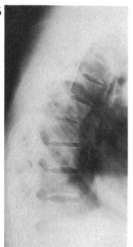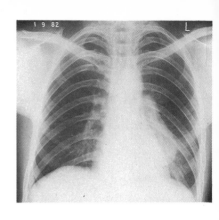

166, 167 A 33-year-old Vietnamese had complained of interscapular pain for 7 months and of a diffuse soft swelling over the L shoulder blade for 2 months. The spine was tender and the L plantar was extensor.
(a) What do the X-rays show?
(b) What is the diagnosis?
(c) Would you advise laminectomy?

168 An elderly patient with headache, malaise, tenderness over the L temple and an ESR of 120.
(a) Would you wait for a biopsy before starting treatment?
(b) What is the starting dose; for how long should it be sustained; is an 'alternate day' regime acceptable?

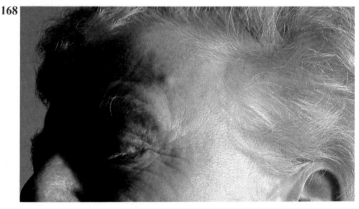

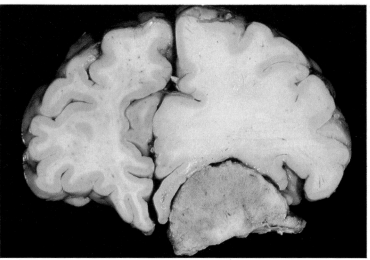

169 A section through the frontal lobes of a patient who presented with fits and a change of personality.
(a) What is the lesion?
(b) What would you look for in addition to frontal lobe signs?
(c) Although classed as 'benign' it is often impossible to resect lesions of this sort. Why?

170 This 17-year-old patient with nocturnal enuresis complained that his tongue was sore.
(a) What is your provisional diagnosis?
(b) To what extent should he be investigated initially?
(c) Under certain domestic circumstances, the patient's life could be at risk. What are they?

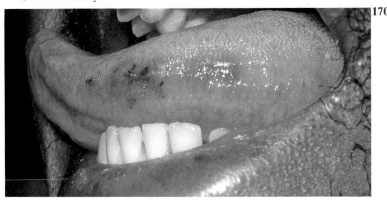

171

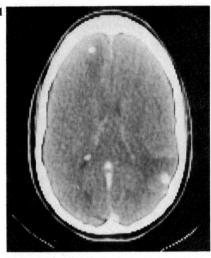

171 A 38-year-old Pakistani presented with fits and headache.
(a) What does this enhanced scan show?
(b) Are such lesions likely to respond to treatment with drugs?
(c) Apart from prescribing appropriate treatment, what else must be done?

172

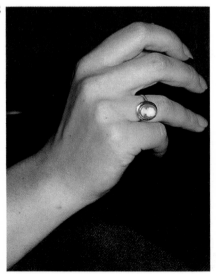

172 A woman developed weakness of the hand after playing table tennis all evening.
(a) What does the posture of the limb suggest?
(b) What is the cause?
(c) Suggest some other causes.

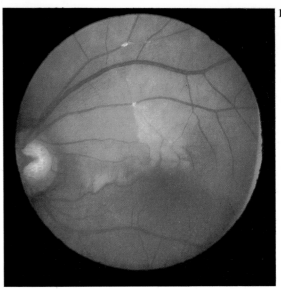

173 Shortly after a road accident in which he sustained a whiplash injury, this patient became hemiplegic.
(a) What is the lesion illustrated?
(b) How was it caused?
(c) Is the delayed onset of the hemiparesis unusual?

174 (a) What abnormality is visible on this film?
(b) What is the differential diagnosis?
(c) How might such a patient present?

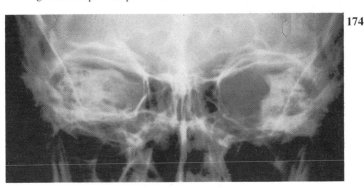

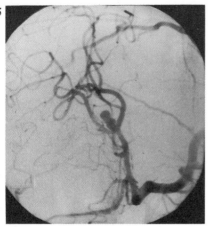

175, 176 These films of a patient thought to have had a subarachnoid haemorrhage were taken shortly after admission.
(a) How do you interpret these findings?
(b) How would you resolve the problem?

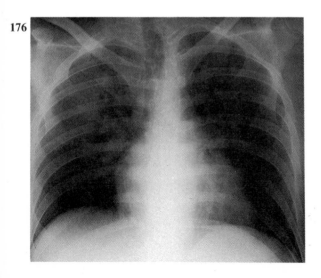

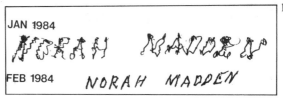

JAN 1984 NORAH MADDEN

FEB 1984 NORAH MADDEN

177 (a) What is the matter with this woman?
(b) Will her hands shake more when they are at rest?
(c) Why has her writing improved?

178 A diagram of a coronal section through the cavernous sinus.
(a) Label A–G.
(b) What effect does an intracavernous aneurysm usually have on vision; facial sensation; the pupil?

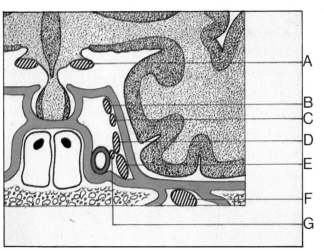

178

A
B
C
D
E
F
G

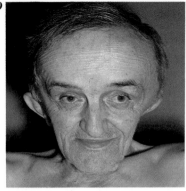

179 (a) What is the diagnosis?
(b) What are the neurological complications
of this condition?

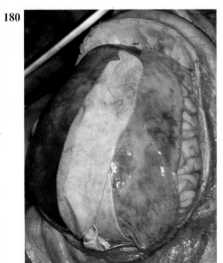

180 (a) What is this lesion?
(b) Name three predispos-
ing factors.
(c) What is the most
common symptom?

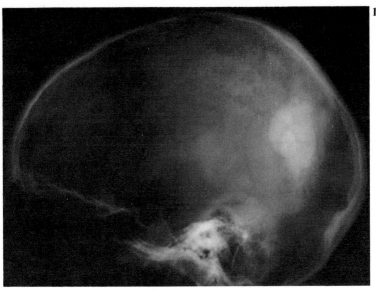

181 (a) What is this lesion?
(b) What would you wish to see?

182 A patient complained of being dazzled by sunlight and oncoming headlights.
(a) What is the likely diagnosis?
(b) What other signs would you expect?
(c) What is the cause?

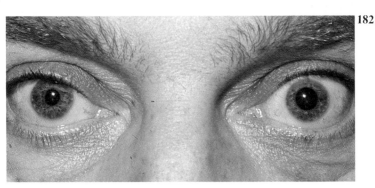

183

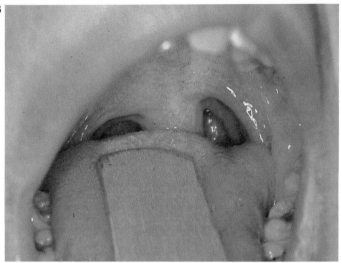

183 (a) What does the appearance of the palate suggest?
(b) Where does the nerve concerned leave the skull?
(c) What other signs does a lesion of this nerve produce?

184 (a) What does this sign indicate?
(b) Where does the nerve leave the skull?
(c) Is it involved in the lateral medullary syndrome?

184

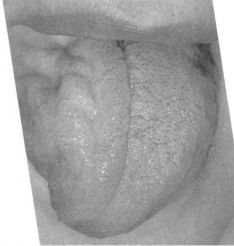

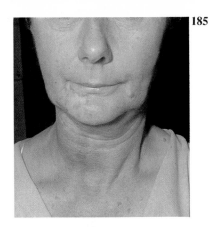

185, 186 (a) What do these illustrations show?
(b) The patient was deaf on the R and had the defects illustrated in **183** and **184**. Where is the lesion?

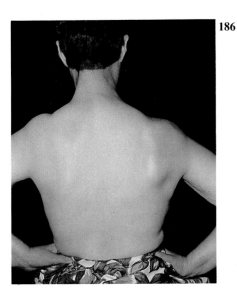

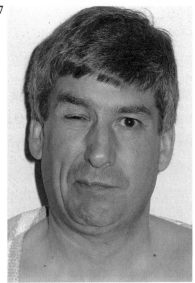

187, 188 A man complained of twitching of the R side of his face.
(a) What do the illustrations show?
(b) What is the cause?
(c) What is the treatment?

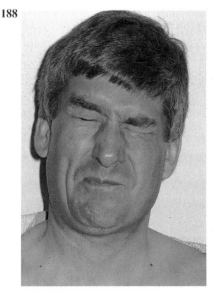

189 This unusual midline 'tumour' had been producing symptoms for 25 years.
(a) What is it?
(b) What signs would confirm the diagnosis?
(c) Explain the patient's complaint that, 'things jump up and down when I look at them'.

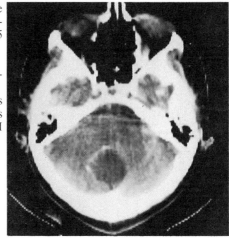

189

190 (a) What is this lesion?
(b) With what is it associated?
(c) What other neurological abnormalities may be found in such patients?

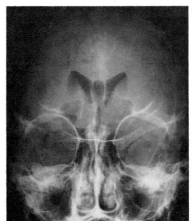

190

191

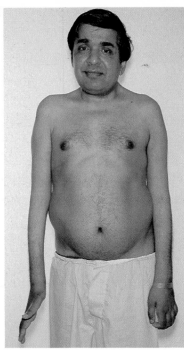

191, 192 This man had extensive fasciculation in the arms.
(a) What is the differential diagnosis?
(b) How do these conditions differ?
(c) What would you hope to see on the definitive investigation?

192

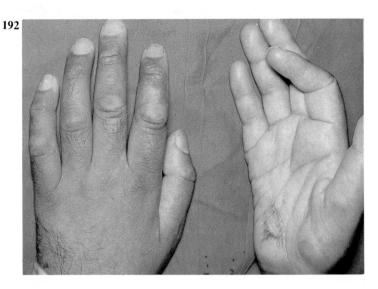

193 A 54-year-old man had recently suffered two nocturnal fits.
(a) What is the lesion?
(b) In what other way do these lesions commonly present?
(c) Is he likely to experience this problem?

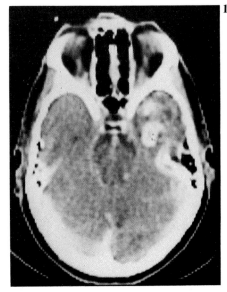

194 A woman presented with headache. What possibilities should be considered?

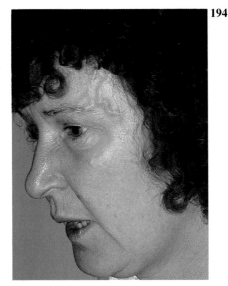

195

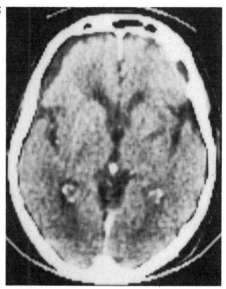

195, 196 Scans of a middle-aged man with dementia, ataxia and poly-neuritis.
(a) What is the main abnormality?
(b) What is the most likely cause?
(c) What causes should be considered if the patient lapsed into coma?

196

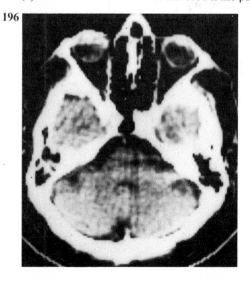

197 (a) What is the matter with this man?
(b) What are the cardinal features of the condition?
(c) In unilateral cases, is the cerebral lesion ipsi- or contralateral?

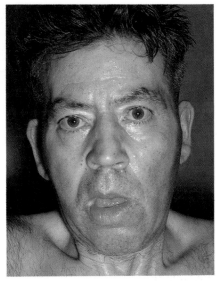

198 (a) What is the abnormality shown?
(b) If you heard a murmur in the head, what diagnosis would you suspect, and what clinical test should be done?

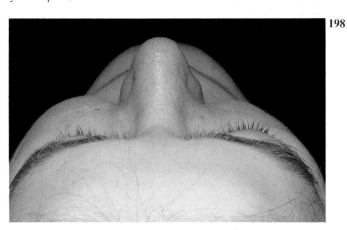

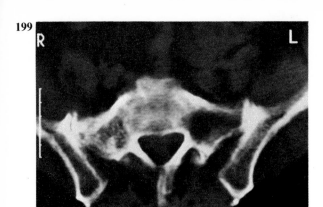

199, 200 CAT scans at S1 and S2 of a patient with a history of rectal carcinoma. Would you expect to find evidence of: (a) weakness; (b) loss of sensation; (c) loss of sphincter control?

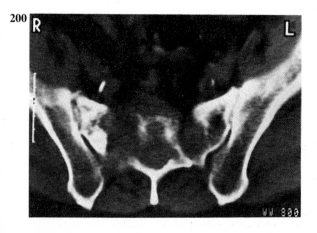

ANSWERS

1, 2 (a) Closing the eyes reveals synkinetic movements on the left and not, as the second picture shows, weakness on the right.
(b) Misdirection of fibres regenerating after injury (note scar). Crocodile tears.
(c) None.

3, 4 (a) Sclerosis or ectopic calcification in the L parietal region and a large globular lesion attached to the vault.
(b) A meningioma.
(c) With evidence of raised intracranial pressure ± fits ± loss of function (especially R inferior quadrantic homonymous hemianopia).

5 (a) He has a R 6th nerve palsy.
(b) The outer one (as always, when the 'bad' eye is covered).
(c) In the absence of other symptoms and signs simply exclude hypertension and diabetes. He is *not* likely to have an aneurysm.

6 (a) The ophthalmic and maxillary divisions of the 5th cranial nerve (note backward extent of V_1).
(b) Fits, ipsilateral ocular defects, contralateral hemiparesis and mental retardation.
(c) Sturge–Weber syndrome — ipsilateral atrophy of and calcification in cerebral cortex (usually posteriorly) ± overlying meningeal angioma.

7 (a) Painless burns due to isoniazid polyneuritis in a patient with erythema ab igne.
(b) Genetically determined failure to metabolise isoniazid, a pyridoxine antagonist.
(c) Retrobulbar neuritis, confusion and convulsions.

8, 9 (a) Virtually none.
(b) Usually at the lower border of L1, but varies from the lower border of T12 to the upper border of L3; one vertebra below adult level; lower border of S2.

10, 11 (a) A hypoplastic foot and an excessive growth of hair in the lumbar region suggest spina bifida occulta.
(b) A dimple in the natal cleft, a palpable defect in the laminae, evidence of a cauda equina lesion, trophic changes in the feet and developmental disorders elsewhere.
(c) Radiological investigation with a view to surgery.

12 (a) A Bjerrum screen to test the central visual field.
(b) A 'hysterical' patient or an incompetent doctor (isoptres, like contour lines, cannot cross).
(c) 'Corkscrew' fields and fields which do not constrict as the patient moves towards the screen.

13 (a) Widening of an intervertebral foramen by a dumb-bell neurofibroma which is not compressing the cord.
(b) Clinically, 8 and 5, but at autopsy they are much more common on 10.

14 (a) Metastases from a malignant melanoma.
(b) With fits or with a subarachnoid haemorrhage.
(c) An appearance like Indian ink.

15 (a) Weakness of external rotation due to paralysis of the R infraspinatus.
(b) Neuralgic amyotrophy.
(c) Good, but recovery may take more than 12 months.

16 (a) A 3rd nerve palsy.
(b) An externally rotated eye with a dilated pupil.
(c) Local lesions (eg inflammation of lid), congenital ptosis, myasthenia gravis, hysterical ptosis and voluntary closure to prevent diplopia.

17 (a) An oblique view showing spondylosis and narrowing of the foramen at C4/5 due to a congenital fusion of C3/4.
(b) Limitation of neck movements, weakness of the shoulder muscles, depression of the biceps jerk, impairment of sensation on the lateral aspect of the arm and a spastic paraplegia.
(c) Vertebrobasilar ischaemia.

18 (a) Ataxia telangiectasia.
(b) A low gamma globulin and a high alpha fetoprotein.
(c) Infection or (? reticulo-endothelial) malignant disease.

19 (a) A 3/second spike and wave discharge.
(b) Absences (*petit mal*).
(c) The EEG abnormality is inherited as a Mendelian dominant, but less than half of those affected will have fits.

20 (a) Cysticercosis.
(b) Residence overseas.
(c) Mental changes, raised intracranial pressure, focal lesions in the brain and cord, meningitis and muscular 'hypertrophy'.

21 (a) A disorder of voluntary muscle which is not secondary to a neurological disorder; a disorder of the spinal cord; a genetically determined degenerative myopathy.
(b) Wasting of the lower part of the pectoral muscles, a slender biceps and a well-preserved deltoid.

22 (a) R Horner's syndrome.
(b) In the intracranial part of the R ocular sympathetic.
(c) Raeder's paratrigeminal syndrome.

23 (a) A perimeter to test the peripheral visual fields.
(b) A lesion in the *left* temporal lobe (fields are charted as seen by the patient).
(c) As it spares the inferior quadrants, the hemianopia is not of itself a contraindication. However, a recent stroke, inattention or the occurrence or possibility of fits would be.

24 (a) Hypotonia.
(b) Tabes dorsalis.
(c) Deafness.

25 (a) A – enlarged lateral ventricle; B – calcified pineal; C – calcified choroid plexus in enlarged posterior horn; D – colloid cyst in third ventricle.
(b) With intellectual impairment, headache (paroxysmal and/or postural) ataxia, drop attacks and periods of loss of consciousness.
(c) Immediate admission for resection.

26 (a) R-sided papilloedema.
(b) Raised intracranial pressure (in which papilloedema is sometimes strikingly asymmetrical) but in particular a subfrontal tumour compressing the left optic nerve (an 'abortive' Foster Kennedy syndrome).
(c) Anosmia.

27 (a) Ankylosing spondylitis.
(b) Susceptibility to trauma and a cauda equina syndrome.
(c) Arachnoid cysts in the lower part of the spinal canal with adhesions.

28 (a) Motor neurone disease and syringomyelia.
(b) In syringomyelia there is a suspended dissociated sensory loss with scarring and loss of arm reflexes. Fasciculation is less evident and widespread.
(c) Peroneal, distal muscular and distal spinal musular atrophy, bilateral ulnar neuropathy (? in the palm) and syphilitic amyotrophy.

29 (a) T10.
(b) Spinal tenderness and/or root pain at the same level.
(c) By damaging a radicular artery which supplies the cord above its point of entry.

30 (a) Partial (focal) seizures with dysphasia arising near the lower part of the L precentral gyrus.
(b) Headache and vomiting, limb symptoms on the R, loss of consciousness and evidence of a primary elsewhere.
(c) In the L frontal lobe there is a large, ill-defined intracerebral lesion with surrounding oedema which is displacing the falx and ventricles to the R; probably a glioma.

31 (a) The ichthyosis suggests Refsum's disease.
(b) Retinal pigmentation, optic atrophy, deafness, ataxia, hypertrophied nerves and a high CSF protein.
(c) Central and peripheral demyelination due to the deposition of phytanic acid.

32 (a) Broad-based triangular slow waves with phase reversal about the R anterior temporal region.
(b) Herpes simplex encephalitis.
(c) Encephalitis is a non-suppurative inflammatory disorder of the brain, commonly generalised but sometimes mainly focal, which causes clouding of consciousness with or without focal signs.

33 (a) Calcification in a dilated ascending aorta.
(b) Serological tests for syphilis.
(c) The L recurrent laryngeal, the L sympathetic and (with a large aneurysm) adjacent nerve roots.

34 (a) Arrested hydrocephalus.
(b) Low I.Q.; spastic paraplegia.
(c) None, unless new symptoms suggest 'decompensation'.

35 (a) Radial nerve.
(b) Compression of the terminal branch by the watch bracelet.
(c) Cheiralgia paraesthetica.

36 (a) A space-occupying lesion outlined by contrast between C1 and C3.
(b) It was a meningioma, but could have been a neurofibroma.
(c) The majority of the ear is supplied by C2/3.

37 (a) Winging of the scapulae; muscular dystrophy.
(b) The pectoral, biceps and brachioradialis muscles (cf **21**).
(c) A neuropathy and a spinal atrophy.

38–41 (a) A R 3rd nerve palsy.
(b) Yes, scleral vessels on the inner canthus move in a clockwise direction on looking down.
(c) The dilated pupil favours compression and, in the absence of other signs, this is likely to be caused by an aneurysm on the posterior communicating artery.

42 (a) Hydrocephalus due to a large low density lesion in the R cerebellar hemisphere — probably a haemangioblastoma.
(b) With (? minimal) evidence of raised intracranial pressure and ataxia.
(c) Other tumours in the brain or cord, retinal, renal, adrenal and pancreatic lesions and polycythaemia.

43 (a) The clinical manifestation of a sudden disorderly discharge of brain cells.
(b) If he is having fits, yes. The EEG, which shows sharp waves in the top 3 leads and phase reversal between 1 and 2 (over the R temporal lobe), is compatible with a diagnosis of partial or focal epilepsy — but you do not treat an EEG.
(c) Forbid driving and look for a focal (? neoplastic) cause.

44, 45 (a) A L lower motor neurone facial palsy (patient cannot furrow brow on that side).
(b) Cotton wool in the ear suggests an acute or chronic pyogenic infection, geniculate herpes or (as proved to be the case) pain due to an infiltrating tumour.

46 (a) A R paraspinal mass two levels below a collapsed thoracic vertebra.
(b) Metastatic disease or myeloma. Inflammation is less likely as the adjacent vertebrae appear to be intact.

47 (a) Numerous plaques of demyelination, many in a typical subcortical or periventricular position.
(b) Lesions in the central nervous system of young adults which are disseminated in space and time.
(c) A slight excess of lymphocytes and protein, a marked increase in the IgG/albumin ratio and oligoclonal bands.

48 (a) Testing near-vision.
(b) To wear his reading glasses and cover one eye.
(c) N5 — a point that may be important if the 'loss of vision' is thought to be hysterical.

49, 50 (a) Multiple fractures with an extradural haematoma (and a less obvious subdural on the R).
(b) Rupture of a meningeal artery by a fracture.
(c) In some series it occurred in less than 50 per cent.

51 (a) A large calcified mass in the left middle fossa, arising from the sphenoid bone.
(b) A meningioma.
(c) Probably with (complex partial or temporal lobe) seizures followed by evidence of raised intracranial pressure.

52 (a) A central scotoma in the L eye of a young woman.
(b) Retrobulbar neuritis.
(c) There will be a substantial or complete recovery of vision, but 50 per cent of those with no previous symptoms will develop multiple sclerosis (usually of a relatively benign type) within 4 years.

53 (a) Bilateral ptosis.
(b) Congenital ptosis, myasthenia gravis, muscular dystrophies, ocular myopathy and syphilis.
(c) The expressionless face and smooth brow favour a dystrophy or myasthenia; the receding hairline and temporalis wasting suggest dystrophia myotonica.

54 (a) Myasthenia gravis; a thymoma.
(b) Yes, because it might be malignant.
(c) Probably not.

55, 56 (a) Tendon xanthomas; hypercholesterolaemia.
(b) Ischaemic heart disease, arthritis and a positive family history.
(c) Yes, in a man under the age of 55 years, but the risk of ischaemic heart disease is much greater.

57 (a) On the L, where the sulci are obliterated, there is a peripheral crescentic shadow — a subdural haematoma.
(b) Venous haemorrhage due to trauma (often trivial) or a coagulation defect.
(c) Depression of consciousness.

58 (a) Wasting of the buttocks.
(b) Diabetic amyotrophy.
(c) A proximal neuropathy which resolves when the diabetes is under good control.

59 (a) A frontal burrhole, air in dilated frontal horns and contrast in the 3rd ventricle, aqueduct and posterior horn.
(b) The sharp angulation of the top of the aqueduct is indicative of a posteriorly placed posterior fossa mass.
(c) Twining's kink.

60 (a) Wasting with atrophy of the fingertips in a coloured patient suggests leprosy.
(b) Thickened nerves and patches of anaesthetic skin.
(c) Tuberculoid.

61, 62 (a) A R lower motor neurone facial palsy.
(b) The patient has a palsy of conjugate gaze to the R, presumably due to a lesion in the pontine centre near the R abducens nucleus — which is surrounded by 7.
(c) Demyelination or a vascular accident.

63–65 (a) An internuclear ophthalmoplegia (R eye adducts on convergence but not on lateral gaze).
(b) In the R medial longitudinal bundle.
(c) A 'one and a half syndrome' — ie loss of conjugate gaze to the R and of adduction on conjugate gaze to the L.

66 (a) i) Yes. ii) Will be decided by subsequent events. A young patient with a penetrating missile injury and early epilepsy runs a very high (greater than 50 per cent) risk of further seizures, but paediatricians are reluctant to prescribe without a definite indication.
(b) A cerebral abscess.

67 (a) A filling defect, probably due to lateral prolapse of the L4/5 disc.
(b) The corresponding root, which can be seen approaching the pedicle above the lesion, is (characteristically) intact. The L5 sheath is obliterated, and the swollen root — along with S1 — is displaced medially.
(c) Weakness of dorsiflexion, numbness on the dorsum of the foot and (possibly) a depressed ankle jerk.

68 (a) (Pneumococcal) meningitis.
(b) Give 1M units of soluble penicillin at once.
(c) No — if only because there might be an abscess.

69, 70 (a) An internal carotid aneurysm in the R cavernous sinus.
(b) R3, 4, ophthalmic and maxillary divisions of 5 and 6.
(c) Probably dilated and fixed, but if the sympathetic fibres are also involved it will be of normal size.

71, 72 (a) Concomitant and paralytic.

(b) In a concomitant squint the angle of deviation of the visual axes is always the same. In a paralytic squint it is greater when the patient fixes with his 'bad' eye.

(c) A concomitant squint appears in infancy in an eye which is often defective. The range of movement is full and the patient rarely complains of diplopia.

73 (a) An aneurysm of the posterior communicating artery.

(b) With a 3rd nerve palsy or a subarachnoid haemorrhage (cf **16, 38–41**).

74 (a) Parkinsonism.

(b) Idiopathic, postencephalitic and drug-induced.

(c) Methylphenyltetrahydropyridine — an impurity in a pethidine analogue, which produces a Parkinsonian syndrome.

75 (a) A cerebellar haemorrhage, probably due to rupture of a micro-aneurysm in a hypertensive patient.

(b) Surgical evacuation.

76 (a) Optic atrophy, almost certainly primary.

(b) A field defect, a defective direct response to light and abnormal evoked responses.

(c) Compression of the optic nerve, as opposed to retrobulbar neuritis.

77 (a) Wasting of the left thenar eminence; compression of the median nerve by the transverse carpal ligament.

(b) The lesion is in a well-manicured left hand; direct trauma to the median nerve, or a cervical rib or band.

78 (a) Upward flow of contrast is blocked by a long posteriorly placed lesion, probably an epidural staphylococcal abscess.

(b) Antibiotics followed at once by laminectomy and drainage.

(c) Lumbar puncture is contraindicated if local sepsis is a possibility.

79 (a) The L hemisphere is swollen and there is haemorrhagic infarction on the L and to a lesser extent on the R, due to sagittal sinus thrombosis.

pressure.

(c) Trauma, meningiomas, infection, sickle cell disease, oral contraceptives and pregnancy.

80 (a) Fat necrosis due to insulin injections.

(b) Diabetics on insulin should not drive vocationally, and all should be well-stabilised and report their disability.

(c) Conviction for driving while under the influence of a drug leads to automatic disqualification for 6 months.

81, 82 (a) A calcified mass opposite L1, the pedicles of which are indistinct. The canal is blocked and the lower border of an ovoid tumour is outlined above the roots of the cauda equina.
(b) A benign intra-arachnoid tumour. The calcification — a rare finding — is almost diagnostic of a meningioma.
(c) Suspected spinal block and suspected thrombosis of the lateral sinus.

83, 84 (a) Myasthenia gravis; injection of edrophonium.
(b) X-ray of mediastinum; tests for anti-acetyl choline receptor and antistriated muscle antibodies; EMG.
(c) Penicillamine.

85 (a) A L carotid arteriogram on which the anterior cerebral and other vessels are stretched round a large mass (? a meningioma) in the upper part of the frontal lobe.
(b) With change of personality, (? adversive) fits and ataxia followed by dysphasia, R hemiparesis and (ultimately) evidence of raised intracranial pressure.
(c) Erosion of the posterior clinoid, hyperostosis, ectopic calcification and enlarged vascular channels.

86 (a) Visuo-spatial agnosia.
(b) The R (non-dominant) parieto-occipital lobe.
(c) Disturbances of cortical sensation (2 point, position, stereognosis, number recognition); inattention; other evidence of L-sided neglect; a field defect.

87 (a) Weakness of muscles in the pelvic girdle.
(b) The patient looks too old to have a Duchenne dystrophy, but might have the benign X-linked (Becker) or limb girdle type or spinal muscular atrophy.

88 (a) Ventriculography (note burrhole, top R).
(b) Suture spread, with massive enlargement of the lateral and third ventricles and the interventricular foramen.
(c) Aqueduct stenosis, a midline tumour, a developmental defect in the posterior fossa or adhesions.

89 (a) Subdural abscess.
(b) Sinus or ear infections, injury to or infection of the skull, and septicaemia.
(c) Cerebral infarction due to thrombophlebitis.

90 (a) Dysgraphia.
(b) An inability to express formed ideas in writing when the ability to write is unimpaired.
(c) Inferior frontal gyrus of the dominant hemisphere.

91 (a) A burrhole, an opacity (catheter tip) above the pituitary fossa and 'Sturge–Weber' tramline calcification over the occiput (cf **66**).
(b) No.
(c) No.

92–97 (a) A crossed hemiparesis (ie with contralateral cranial neuropathy) and an internuclear ophthalmoplegia both indicate a brainstem lesion. It originated near the R facial nucleus in the pons.
(b) Bilateral facial weakness and paralysis of horizontal gaze. Vertical gaze and convergence are normal. This is a bilateral version of the lesion seen in **61** and **62**.
(c) A young woman with bilateral internuclear ophthalmoplegia of gradual onset usually has demyelination.

98 (a) A large haematoma in the R hemisphere.
(b) Rupture of a microaneurysm which, as is occasionally the case, was subcortical rather than capsular.
(c) Surgical evacuation. Such patients often make a good recovery, possibly because fibres are separated and compressed but not destroyed.

99, 100 (a) Enquire whether his job depends upon writing and whether, for all other purposes, his hand is 'normal'; writer's cramp.
(b) Psychosomatic.
(c) Re-education, relaxation techniques and behavioural therapy.

101 (a) Ophthalmic zoster.
(b) Injury to the eye from corneal scarring or panophthalmitis (said to be less common when, as here, the territory of the nasociliary branch is spared) and postherpetic neuralgia.
(c) The varicella virus — sometimes activated by local lesions irritating nerve roots, immunosuppressive therapy or systemic infections.

102 (a) A midline mass indenting the posterior end of the 3rd ventricle and hydrocephalus.
(b) A pinealoma.
(c) With evidence of raised intracranial pressure, defective vertical and convergent gaze, pupillary abnormalities, ataxia and (occasionally in boys) precocious development.

103 (a) Spina bifida occulta (same case as **10** and **11**).
(b) Defective closure of the neural tube and/or vertebral canal with incomplete separation from surface ectoderm. Hydromyelia, and tethering, compression or transection of the cord by bands, dermoids, lipomas or diastematomyelia.
(c) Yes, about tenfold.

104 (a) Cavernous sinus thrombosis.
(b) Spread to the R cavernous sinus.
(c) Relapses are common, and antibiotics must be given for 2 or 3 months.

105, 106 (a) A L C8/T1 radiculopathy due to a lesion in the canal.
(b) In **106** the shoulders are pulled down to reveal erosion of the C7 spine.
(c) Tuberculosis.

107 (a) Paralysis of ocular movements, facial and bulbar muscles.
(b) The Miller–Fisher variant of acute infective polyneuritis.
(c) Many have an encephalitis in addition to the inflammatory polyneuritis.

108 (a) Heart block.
(b) Insertion of a pacemaker.

109 (a) Stenosis at the carotid bifurcation, with slowing of the intracranial circulation.
(b) Diminished carotid pulsation with a bruit, attacks of impairment of vision in the ipsilateral eye and contralateral long tract signs.
(c) 3 per cent.

110 (a) Meralgia paraesthetica (compression of the lateral cutaneous nerve of the thigh).
(b) Numbness over the whole of the anterolateral aspect of one or (occasionally) both thighs.

111 (a) von Recklinghausen's disease.
(b) Diffuse neurofibroma formation in the terminal branches of nerve fibres, often associated with proliferation or hypertrophy of adjacent tissues (elephantiasis neuromatosa).
(c) Optic atrophy, glaucoma, glioma of the optic nerve, and compression or raised pressure due to a neurofibroma, meningioma or glioma.

112 (a) Thinning of the posterior clinoid process and a double floor in the pituitary fossa suggest a pituitary adenoma.
(b) Headache, over- and/or undersection of pituitary hormones, bitemporal hemianopia and optic atrophy.
(c) Hypogonadism.

113–116 (a) A partial L 3rd nerve palsy (little ptosis and a pupil of normal size — cf **16** and **38–41**). The 6th nerve (abduction) is intact.
(b) Ischaemia or diabetes (compression usually causes pupillary dilatation by damaging the superficially placed parasympathetic fibres).

117 (a) Peroneal muscular atrophy.
(b) Usually by dominant inheritance.
(c) A hypertrophic demyelinating neuropathy; an axonal neuropathy; a form due to degeneration of the anterior horn cells.

118–121 (a) Hemifacial atrophy.
(b) Some cases are attributed to scleroderma, and the patient may have a groove (*'coup de sabre'*) on the skull. Others are associated with conditions that damage the cervical sympathetic system. Most are unexplained.
(c) Transplantation of adipose tissue to minimise deformity.

122, 123 (a) A large, irregular tumour deeply situated in the R hemisphere—a malignant glioma.
(b) Not with such a large lesion that has developed so rapidly.
(c) If his mental state does not render him unfit to drive, the risk of having a seizure does so.

124 (a) 1 – auricular branch, 2 – chorda tympani, 3 – nerve to stapedius, 4 – greater superficial petrosal, 5 – nervus intermedius, 6 – geniculate ganglion.
(b) 1 – involvement in geniculate herpes may produce rash in ear; 2 and 3 – loss of taste and hyperacusis in Bell's palsy indicate a lesion in the petrous temporal, which is likely to be severe.

125 (a) A Charcot or neuropathic joint.
(b) Tabes dorsalis, syringomyelia and diabetes.
(c) Impaired sensation, hypotonia and trauma.

126 (a) Unequal dilated pupils, and defects in convergence/accommodation and the reaction to light.
(b) Tumours, vascular accidents and encephalitis in the region of the superior colliculi.
(c) By asking the patient to fix on a static object and tilting the head forwards.

127–130 (a) 1 and 8 – lateral spinothalmic tract; 2 and 6 – medial lemniscus/posterior column; 3 – 9th, 10th and 11th cranial nerves; 4 – 12th cranial nerve; 5 and 7 – pyramidal tract.
(b) In the pons.
(c) **127**: posterior inferior cerebellar artery thrombosis; **128**: hemisection of the cord due to trauma tumour infarction or demyelination; **129**: anterior spinal artery thrombosis; **130**: syringomyelia.
(d) Dissociated sensory loss.
(e) Dysphagia, dysphonia, and ipsilateral ataxia, Horner's syndrome and facial numbness.

131 (a) Dermatomyositis.
(b) Subcutaneous calcification.
(c) Not below the age of 40 years.

132 (a) L frontal abscess surrounded by oedema.
(b) Sinusitis, trauma, pulmonary infections, endocarditis and congenital heart disease.
(c) No; even the suspicion of an abscess is an absolute contraindication.

133 (a) Inability to 'pinch' with the R thumb and index due to weakness of the deep flexors.
(b) If this is the only sign in the hand, the patient has a lesion in the anterior interosseous branch of the median nerve, probably due to neuralgic amyotrophy. (Same patient as **15**.)

134 (a) Pseudomeningoceles, due to a severe traction injury to the brachial plexus.
(b) An anaesthetic flail arm.
(c) Horner's syndrome, paralysis of rhomboids and serratus anterior, paraspinal anaesthesia and preservation of triple response and sensory conduction, which indicate an (untreatable) proximal lesion.

135, 136 (a) Hyperostosis of the sphenoid in front of the pituitary fossa (which is not enlarged), and an adjacent mass.
(b) Pituitary tumours, craniopharyngiomas, aneurysms and meningiomas. Hyperostosis suggests a meningioma.
(c) With visual failure, optic atrophy, a (? bitemporal) field defect and fits.

137, 138 (a) Raised intracranial pressure, possibly (in view of irregular periods and appearance) due to benign intracranial hypertension.
(b) A CAT scan to exclude a tumour and hydrocephalus, followed by a lumbar puncture.
(c) Endocrine disorders (adrenal, thyroid, parathyroid and ovarian), vitamin A, tetracycline, thrombosis of venous sinuses.

139, 140 (a) Facial diplegia with ptosis (which is *not* due to a 7th nerve palsy) — Möbius' syndrome.
(b) Weakness of the external ocular muscles and tongue, club foot, malformations of the arm and mental deficiency.
(c) Rarely.

141 (a) A lacune in the R internal capsule.
(b) Occlusion of a perforating branch of the middle cerebral artery in a hypertensive patient.
(c) With pure motor or pure sensory hemiplegia, homolateral cerebellar ataxia and pyramidal tract signs or (in the pons) the 'dysarthria/clumsy hand' syndrome.

142 (a) Destruction of the proximal part of the L 2nd rib.
(b) A metastasis or a Pancoast's tumour.
(c) The cervical sympathetic and the lower roots of the brachial plexus.

143 (a) A – basilar artery, B – superior cerebellar artery, C – posterior cerebral artery, D – oculomotor nerve, E – posterior communicating artery, F – internal carotid artery.
(b) The L 3rd nerve is compressed by the (herniated) temporal lobe.
(c) A fixed dilated L pupil.

144 (a) Wedging with preservation of the disc spaces suggests trauma or neoplastic infiltration as opposed to tubercle.
(b) Loss of the ankle jerks, saddle anaesthesia and retention.
(c) Damage to the sacral roots of the cauda equina, which occupy a vulnerable central position in the lumbosacral spine.

145 (a) Tract A: from midline 'centres' for convergence and vertical gaze beneath the colliculi (cf **102** and **126**); Tract B: from centres for conjugate lateral gaze in the opposite hemisphere.
(b) The medial longitudinal bundle. An internuclear ophthalmoplegia, with failure of the L eye to adduct on lateral gaze. Convergence is normal. (The shaded area indicates the site of the lesion in **61–65**, which would involve the R medial longitudinal bundle.)

146–148 (a) Ectopic calcification, mainly in the basal ganglia.
(b) The patient may have hypoparathyroidism, pseudohypoparathyroidism or a familial disorder sometimes associated with dementia, ataxia and extrapyramidal signs.

149 (a) Apathy, drowsiness, amnesia, ataxia and fits.
(b) Symptomatically (ie with analgesics, anticonvulsants, antidepressants, steroids, etc).
(c) A biopsy track.

150 (a) Abductor pollicis brevis.
(b) Median nerve.
(c) Opponens pollicis.

151 (a) Palsies of 3 and the ophthalmic division of 5 on the L (ptosis, loss of adduction, ? dilated pupil and sensory loss).
(b) An aneurysm in the cavernous sinus.
(c) Palsies of L4 and 6.

152 (a) Hypertrophy of the musculo-cutaneous nerve.
(b) A family history of polyneuritis.
(c) In any recurrent or protracted demyelinating neuropathy.

153 (a) Winging of the scapula; damage to the long thoracic nerve by injuries to the shoulder, direct surgical trauma or neuralgic amyotrophy.
(b) An accessory nerve palsy; the sternomastoid and trapezius are wasted, the upper angle of the scapula moves away from the midline, and when the arms are extended it rotates downwards and winging decreases.

154 (a) Coarsening of the features, due to phenytoin.
(b) No.
(c) Other connective tissue disorders include gum hypertrophy, a lupus-like syndrome and Dupuytren's contracture.

155 (a) Hydrocephalus, and a large spherical lesion between the frontal lobes which has a discrete nodule at one point on the wall.
(b) A giant aneurysm which will probably present with fits, personality change or evidence of chiasmal compression, but may eventually rupture.

156, 157 (a) Severe bilateral ptosis, with a furrowed brow and normal facial movements.
(b) Bilateral ptosis with furrowing is seen in tabes and congenital ptosis, but is rarely as severe. A bilateral 3rd nerve palsy must be considered (cf **53**).

158–160 (a) Paralysis of adduction (which was bilateral) and of vertical gaze; slight dilatation of the L pupil.
(b) In the centre for vertical gaze in the dorsum of the midbrain and/or in the 3rd nerve nuclei.
(c) The most rostral part — the Edinger Westphal nucleus — because the pupils are barely affected.

161 (a) Multiple nodules involving the roots of the cauda equina, outlined at myelography.
(b) Metastatic tumours, or possibly neurofibromas.

162, 163 (a) The posterior tibial nerves have been ligated.
(b) Occasionally, in advanced cases.

164 (a) The calcified pineal is displaced to the R.
(b) When it is more than 3 mm from the midline.
(c) Supratentorially in the posterior two-thirds of the skull on the L.

165 (a) Superficial enhancement in the R frontoparietal region.
(b) A cerebral infarct.
(c) After the 2nd week, for about a month.

166, 167 (a) A slight kyphosis with narrowing of a thoracic disc space, erosion of the adjacent vertebrae and a retro-pleural abscess.
(b) Pott's disease of the spine.
(c) Surgical treatment is required because there is an abscess which threatens to point and evidence of cord damage. Laminectomy should be avoided because the lesion is anterior and the stability of the spine may depend upon the integrity of the neural arches.

168 (a) Treatment of cranial arteritis is urgent and will not interfere with a biopsy performed soon afterwards.
(b) A minimum of 60 mg prednisolone daily for at least 2 weeks; an 'alternate day' regime is unacceptable.

169 (a) A subfrontal meningioma.
(b) Anosmia, optic atrophy and hyperostosis (cf **26** and **135**).
(c) Because of size, position, infiltration of bone or the sagittal sinus, and malignant degeneration.

170 (a) A nocturnal seizure with a characteristic bite on the side of the tongue.
(b) If there are no other symptoms and no signs, an EEG and skull X-ray would suffice.
(c) Patients who have seizures while asleep occasionally aspirate blood or vomit—especially when drunk; snoozing in the bath can be lethal.

171 (a) Nodules surrounded by oedema in the L frontal and R parietal regions — probably tuberculomas.
(b) Yes.
(c) Notification, and the patient should be warned that he must not drive.

172 (a) Paralysis of the extensors of the fingers and the extensor ulnaris (but not radialis) by a posterior interosseous nerve lesion.
(b) Repeated trauma to the nerve as it traverses the supinator.
(c) Lipomas, fractures and prolonged use of a screwdriver.

173 (a) Numerous cholesterol emboli with an area of retinal infarction.
(b) Indirect trauma to an atheromatous carotid artery.
(c) In nearly 50 per cent of cases it appears 10 hours or more after the injury.

174 (a) Erosion of the L petrous temporal bone.
(b) Acoustic neurofibroma, epidermoid, trigeminal neuroma, meningioma, chordoma or metastasis.
(c) With symptoms and signs of damage to the 8th and 5th cranial nerves, followed by raised intracranial pressure and a cerebellar deficit.

175, 176 (a) The patient could have pneumonia or the adult respiratory distress syndrome secondary to a subarachnoid haemorrage. Conversely, he might have pneumococcal or tuberculous meningitis, the aneurysm being an incidental finding.
(b) Examination of the CSF, preferably after a CAT scan.

177 (a) Essential tremor (cf **74**).
(b) No
(c) She has probably been given propranolol or alcohol.

178 (a) A – II, B – III, C – IV, D – V_1, E – V_2, F – V_3, G – VI.
(b) None; impaired over V_1 and possibly V_2 but *not* V_3; usually dilated due to damage to parasympathetic in III, but if sympathetic is also damaged (in carotid plexus or V_1) it will be of normal size (cf **69, 70** and **151**).

179 (a) Paget's disease.
(b) Headache, fits, platybasia, hydrocephalus, cerebellar signs, cranial nerve palsies and cord compression.

180 (a) Subdural haematoma (cf **57**).
(b) Old age; alcoholism; anticoagulants.
(c) Headache.

181 (a) A tightly-woven plait of hair — a diagnosis which cannot be made from this film alone.
(b) A tangential view, which would show that the 'lesion' is outside the skull.

182 (a) A myotonic (Holmes–Adie) pupil.
(b) Loss of ankle jerks and response to light, with slow and excessive response to accommodation.
(c) Unopposed action of sympathetic due to degeneration of ciliary ganglion.

183 (a) A right vagus palsy.
(b) Through the jugular foramen.
(c) A husky voice and a 'bovine' cough, due to paralysis of a vocal cord.

184 (a) A lower motor neurone lesion of the R 12th cranial nerve.
(b) The anterior condylar foramen.
(c) No. Like the pyramid and the medial lemniscus, it is medially situated (see **127**).

185, 186 (a) Wasting of the sternomastoid, drooping of the shoulder and winging of the scapula on the R. The scapula is rotated downwards, indicating that the trapezius is paralysed and the serratus anterior is unopposed. An accessory nerve palsy (cf **153**).
(b) Along the R side of the brainstem — it proved to be a glomus jugulare tumour.

187, 188 (a) R hemifacial spasm with (characteristic) R facial weakness.
(b) 'Idiopathic'; compression of the nerve by vascular loops, adhesions or (rarely) slowly growing tumours; occasionally follows Bell's palsy; *not* 'psychiatric'.
(c) Injections, partial section of the nerve and faciohypoglossal anastomosis have been replaced by operations to decompress the nerve in the posterior fossa.

189 (a) A dermoid.
(b) A sinus over and/or a defect in the occipital bone in the midline.
(c) She had vertical nystagmus which is commonly associated with lesions near the foramen magnum.

190 (a) Cavitation of the septum pellucidum.
(b) Boxing.
(c) Impairment of intellect and personality, dysarthria, tremor and ataxia.

191, 192 (a) Motor neurone disease and syringomyelia. Both cause weakness and wasting, but the scars on the puffy ('succulent') hand favour syringomyelia.
(b) Syringomyelia runs a longer course, and is associated with scoliosis, nystagmus, loss of arm reflexes and a suspended dissociated sensory loss.
(c) Myelography may show a widened cord and canal, descent of the cerebellar tonsils and (with scanning) contrast in the cavity.

193 (a) An arteriovenous malformation.
(b) A subarachnoid haemorrhage.
(c) About 25 per cent of those presenting with fits will subsequently bleed, and 10 per cent will die of this complication.

194 The patient is not elderly, and the numerous prominent vessels (which look like veins) extend on to the upper part of the orbit. Possible causes are sagittal sinus thrombosis or a vascular tumour of skull, but not cranial arteritis.

195, 196 (a) Gross cerebral and cerebellar atrophy.
(b) Alcohol.
(c) Intoxication, trauma (especially a subdural), ingestion of other drugs, Wernicke's encephalopathy, hepatic coma, hypoglycaemia and water intoxication.

197 (a) Parkinson's disease.
(b) Akinesia, resting tremor and plastic and cogwheel rigidity.
(c) Contralateral.

198 (a) R-sided exophthalmos.
(b) Carotico-cavernous fistula; carotid compression.

199, 200 (a) Probably not, although the lesion in the L ala at S1 might impair plantar flexion.
(b) Yes — saddle anaesthesia, for at S2 the canal and both alae are involved.
(c) Yes — retention with overflow and loss of rectal and urethral sensation.

Index